The Well-Being Handbook

An ... Healing

Cissi Williams

BSc (Hons) Ost. Med. DO, ND, MRN

First published by Findhorn Press in 2005

ISBN 1-84409-053-1

British Library Cataloguing-in-Publication Data.
A catalogue record for this book is available
from the British Library.

Edited by Shari Mueller
Cover design by Damian Keenan
Interior design by Thierry Bogliolo
Printed and bound by WS Bookwell, Finland

Published by
Findhorn Press
305a The Park, Findhorn
Forres IV36 3TE
Scotland, UK
tel 01309 690582/fax 690036
info@findhornpress.com
www.findhornpress.com

Table of Contents

Part VI   Conditions   71

Part VII Therapies 191

Bibliography and References 199

Part I

Well-being Overview

Foreword

This book may not be for everyone, because it requires you to take complete responsibility for your own thoughts, actions, emotions and well-being. However, it will help you to realise that you are the cause of everything that happens in your life, and that only **you** have the power to change yourself and the way you relate to the world. As you change on the inside, everything will change on the outside, because everything you perceive in the outside world is only a projection of your inner world, which is made up of your beliefs, values and past experiences.

So if you are ready to change and embrace life to the fullest, read this book and follow the coaching programme, which will guide you to find out what is stopping you from experiencing complete physical, emotional, mental and spiritual well-being. It will enable you to re-balance your mind, re-energise your body and re-discover your spiritual self, by taking you on an inner journey where you release old negative emotions, such as anger, sadness, fear and guilt; let go of old limiting beliefs and decisions you have about yourself and your life; and guide you to fully forgive yourself and others for past perceived hurts and wrong-doings. By doing these things you will free yourself completely from the past so that you are able to live your life to the fullest in the here and now. This programme will also teach you how to solve difficult problems, manifest solutions and goals in your life, and connect with your inner wisdom.

If you are currently experiencing any of the common conditions covered in the **Conditions** section of this book, I suggest you follow the advice under the specific condition and then do the whole coaching programme. Always trust your inner intuition and do what feels right for you, especially when it comes to the suggested **Therapies**. This will totally transform your health and aid you in achieving and maintaining perfect well-being.

So what will you choose? Will you blame others or circumstances for the way your life is and give your power away? Or will you open your mind to the possibility that perhaps you create your own reality and well-being through your thoughts, actions, perceptions, beliefs and values, and as you change these you completely transform yourself and your life? If you do the latter, then I welcome you to take charge of your life, empower yourself, and join me on this inner journey towards perfect well-being for life.

Introduction

What is perfect well-being? This is a question many have asked and few have truly understood. Some search for the feeling of well-being in their looks or in their physical strength. Others think it is to be found in how much money they make or in their partner or friends. Yet others look for it in status and power. So what is well-being? Is it your looks, your partner or your money? Or is it robust health—when you have managed to go through a winter without getting a cold? It is so much more than any of these things! It is when you are in that place within yourself where **you** reside, where you feel completely connected to **all that is**. To put it simply, well-being is when you are in alignment with the physical, emotional, mental and spiritual aspects of yourself.

"Yeah, right," I can hear you say. "That's not easy to do." The fact is, it is easy to do. Most people think that perfect well-being is such a far-fetched goal, that it is not worth even trying to get there. They continue to lead the same life they have always led, because at least they know they are good at that. To those of you who feel this way, I just want to ask one question, "Is it making you happy?" If not, then what have you got to lose? Wouldn't it be worth at least trying to open up to the possibility that perhaps there is another way?

How can I be so sure that there is another way? Because I have walked it. Many years ago, I had my own 'dark night of the soul' experience. I had a very difficult childhood where I had been abused, and after I left home at age eighteen, I continued to abuse myself. At age twenty-four, living in London, I felt I was all alone in the world and that absolutely no one loved me; I was severely depressed. All the relationships in my life were in an utter mess and my body was in poor health…a reflection of my internal state. The worst, however, was the depression. I felt as if the only solution to my problems was to leave this physical existence and I truly believed no one would miss me.

Then one night I dreamt I saw myself hanging dead in my room, and when I awoke the next morning I realised that the way I was—the way I thought and behaved—did not work. I needed help and fast. I prayed to someone or something to show me the way. At first, nothing seemed to happen. Then I got a strong feeling that I should go home to Stockholm, and two days later I found myself walking around the streets of my beautiful hometown. I was being pulled in a certain direction and I soon found myself standing outside an esoteric bookshop called Vattumannen (The Aquarian). Without knowing what I was looking for, I went inside and felt drawn to pick up three books: *Creative Visualisations, The Power is Within You* and *Love Is the Answer*. As I started reading, I realised that my prayers were being answered. These three books gave me valuable tools for helping me get better. In time, my depression went away and I found my path back to life. Through this I realised that I was meant to help others find their path back to perfect physical, emotional, mental and spiritual well-being. I began studying osteopathy, cranial osteopathy, naturopathy, Pilates, Neuro-Linguistic Programming (NLP), timeline therapy®, hypnosis, healing and various other esoteric studies.

Once I realised I had my own internal power to affect my thoughts and emotions, I never stopped changing. When I hit a stumbling block, be it in the form of physical, emotional, mental or spiritual pain, I never hesitated to look at it, deal with it, and when necessary, ask for help in releasing it.

The results have been amazing—I now lead a totally different life. I am very happily married, with two adorable daughters, and I work with something I absolutely love—helping others find their path back to perfect well-being so that they can be more of who they truly are and share more of their authentic selves with the world. I know from personal experience that it is possible to change, and as you change, you feel more alive, more at peace, and once again filled with an inner joy.

This book is an attempt to share with you what I have learned, so that you, too, can empower yourself to be all that you desire. It requires you to take complete responsibility for your own well-being and happiness, so if you are willing to leave your comfort zone and are prepared to change and take action, then read on. Realise that in order to find your path back to inner happiness and joy, you need to look at and learn from what is stopping you from fully experiencing perfect well-being on every level.

If you have pain or discomfort somewhere, pay attention to it and do something about it. Remember, what you resist persists, and what you look at disappears.

chapter 1

Achieving Perfect Well-Being

How can you achieve this state of inner well-being and happiness? First, you need to remember that you are capable of experiencing this state, because you have felt it before, a long time ago. Don't you have a vague memory of being in a place where you were so at peace, so full of life and joy, that everything was perfect just as it was? Don't you feel a longing to reach that place again? Haven't you tried many times to do just that? Where does that feeling come from?

Before you take on a physical existence you are pure spirit, filled with love, joy and peace, and when you leave your physical existence, you go back to this place. However, when you are here on earth you maintain this place deep within you. It is the place where you are in direct connection with your spiritual self. Here you feel happy, peaceful, radiant, full of energy and with the knowledge that everything is perfect just as it is. It is the place you go every time you feel or give unconditional love. Love is the most powerful and healing force there is—it brings us into direct contact with our true essence, our spiritual self.

To a child, the gateway to this place is often open, which is why children have the ability to enjoy the moment, to be happy for the sake of happiness. A child smiles about 400 times a day, while an adult smiles only about 15 times a day.

What happened? Over time the gate starts to shut, and eventually it may close altogether, so that the inner place where perfect well-being and happiness is a reality, becomes a vague and distant memory.

Opening the gate to your inner happiness

Science now knows that the emotional and mental state has a direct effect on physical health, so when the gate to inner happiness and joy closes, you have set up a fertile ground for 'dis-ease' to develop. What would happen if you were to re-open this gate? And more importantly, how do you do that?

When you find this inner place of perfect happiness again, your body and mind will automatically become more aligned, which brings about health in your whole being. This is not something strange or unnatural, it is what your body is striving toward every second of every day. For every breath you take, every beat of your heart, your body is constantly striving to express more of the life force within, so that you can experience more of life. Even when 'dis-ease' has manifested, the body still tries to heal, and it continues to do so until it finally loses the battle, which is expressed as physical death. Up until that point, providing there is enough energy left, the body will try to be as healthy as possible, and it is very grateful for any assistance it can get. This is where you ask yourself, "How do I open the gate?"

Because you are all such unique and complex individuals, there are many ways to open the gate. You have a physical body but you also have an emotional, mental and spiritual aspect to your being, and you can open the gate through any of these aspects. The key is to find out what caused the gate to shut, and once that is established, to work on all four aspects so that your whole being becomes completely re-aligned with itself. When this re-alignment happens, the gate fully re-opens and you can allow your inner peace, happiness and joy to permeate through all the layers of your being, creating perfect well-being.

Taking responsibility

In the search for the true cause of the gate closing, it is essential to take full responsibility for your own health and well-being. Unfortunately, many people do not want to do this. They feel it is much easier to believe that a 'dis-ease' just happens or that others cause them to feel angry or sad and it has nothing to do with them. If you hold on to this belief, you give your power away to the external world, because you believe there is nothing YOU can do to fully open the gate again.

If you believe that you create your own health and your own reality through your thoughts, actions, beliefs and values, then you can do something about it. This empowers you to take action and to be responsible for your own well-being.

However, just as it is important not to blame others for what is happening in your life, it is also important not to blame yourself. If you fall into the trap of blaming and punishing yourself for what has happened, then you allow yourself

to use your power to attack YOU. This effectively stops you from moving forward in life. Instead, look at yourself and your life, see how you have created your reality through how you choose to perceive it, and look for the wisdom that every difficult experience is bringing to you. Remember that life brings sorrows and joys to everyone, but you are the only person who chooses how you react to what is happening in your life.

What is 'dis-ease'?

The orthodox western medical view sometimes supports the belief that 'dis-ease' is something that just seems to happen, and the way they often try to bring the body back into health is by treating the symptoms of the 'dis-ease', rather than the true cause. Often patients want this, too. Say, for instance, you are suffering with a headache, which seems to linger on for a few days or even weeks. What do you do? Do you take painkillers, which will stop the pain signals reaching the brain and some muscle-relaxants, which will help relax unspecific muscle groups throughout your body? Or do you try to understand what is causing the headache in the first place? Are you stressed about something which is making you tense your muscles in your upper back and neck, leading to restrictions of various joints, which in turn decreases the blood flow to the brain leading to a tension headache? Perhaps you have been carrying something heavy, like a rucksack or a toddler, which has upset the balance of your back and neck, leading to musculo-skeletal dysfunction? Have you had some dental work done recently? Is there something you have been eating or drinking which your body is reacting against? Or maybe the headache is allowing you some rest from an emotional situation you want to avoid dealing with?

Looking into these possibilities is truly trying to find the real cause of the pain. Taking painkillers is just masking the symptoms for the time being, and often the pain will keep coming back with more and more intensity until 'dis-ease' eventually may develop.

The holistic view of 'dis-ease'

Health is your natural way of being. It is the state where your physical, emotional, mental and spiritual aspects are in alignment—the inner place where perfect well-being exists.

What causes you to experience discomfort, pain and 'dis-ease'? It stems from an imbalance in this alignment and the main problem may lie in any of the four areas. Most complementary therapies are structured in such a way that the whole person is addressed and the root cause of the problem can be found. This means that the symptoms merely act as a guide to establish what is truly going on. Most therapies would not want to suppress these symptoms with unnatural methods, such as painkillers, since this valuable guide would then be distorted. Although therapies will vary in their diagnosis and treatment methods, most of them share the same aim, which is to support the healing capacity of the body and the mind through natural means.

Healthy values

There are several avenues you can take if you are serious about achieving and maintaining well-being. First of all you need to make the decision that you, yourself, are responsible for how you feel and for how you experience your life. This is because you only perceive your outer reality according to your inner reality, which is made up of your beliefs, values, and past experiences.

How does this work? You have about 2 million 'bits' per second coming from the external world into your central nervous system. If you were able to perceive all of this, you would most likely go mad. Therefore, you have this inner screening system (beliefs, values and past experiences) which filters out everything except about 134 bits per second, out of which you are only consciously aware of about 7 bits per second (+/-2). This is why when ten people experience the same scenario at exactly the same time you will get ten different accounts of what actually happened. Consequently, your experience is always uniquely your own, and it only has the meaning which you attach to it.

If you do not like what you experience in your life, then change your inner screening system. How do you do that? First you need to discover your values and beliefs for each of the following areas in your life:

- health and fitness
- family
- relationships
- work and career
- personal growth
- spirituality

Start with the area where you are experiencing the most difficulties. Perhaps you have a great career but you have problems with relationships. Write down at least ten values that are important to you about relationships. Then rank them from 1 to 10 in order of importance, one being the most important and ten being the least important. Then ask yourself, "Why is value X important to me?" Write down your answer.

When you look at what is important to you about relationships, you may find that some of your values do not support you in experiencing happiness with a partner. Perhaps one of your values was 'love' and when you asked, "Why is love important to me?" you may have answered, "Because I never felt loved as a child." This indicates that you have an 'away from' value (your internal representation of love is an image of you never feeling loved as a child, and you are moving 'away from' that).

Someone else may also have love as a value and when asked why, she may reply, "Because that is what everything is based on…love is all there is." Her internal representation is a picture of complete love, so she is moving toward it. She has a 'toward' value.

Assign a percentage from 1 to 100 of how much your value is 'away from' or 'toward' for you. You may say it is 80% 'away from' and 20% 'toward'. This gives you a very clear indication that you have some issues relating to love that you need to look at and deal with.

Given that information, which one of these two different values do you think will produce a healthy attitude toward relationships and result in a happy relationship? That's right, the 'toward' value. Why? Because you get what you focus on. 'Away from' values take up a lot of energy, because the negative internal representation—which is being fed to your central nervous system—creates inner tension and conflict.

Look at your values again and ask yourself, "How much are each of these an 'away from' or 'toward' value for me?" Write the percentage down next to each value. Then take a good look at your list of values. Are they supporting you in your goal of being happy and well?

What limiting beliefs have you formed that are causing you to have the 'away from' values that you have? For example, the person with the 80% 'away from' value of love, may have an underlying limiting belief of "I am unlovable."

What are the limiting beliefs that have caused your 'away from' values? Be really honest with yourself and make a list of your limiting beliefs.

Follow the same process for all the main areas of your life that you listed. Make sure you write down all the limiting beliefs and decisions which have formed your 'away from' values. Later in the book you will go back to your list of values, so keep them for future reference. In the coaching programme you will be given meditation exercises for releasing negative emotions, limiting beliefs and decisions, which will have a dramatic impact on your present values. It will release your 'away from' values, and you will be left with all your values being 100% 'toward'.

Releasing negative emotions

This is of utmost importance. It is impossible to be healthy and happy when you harbour negative emotions, such as anger, sadness, fear, guilt, hurt and depression. We will go through detailed meditation exercises for releasing these emotions. I strongly encourage you to do them. When you release negative emotions you are able to feel love and compassion for yourself and others. This frees you to fully be the person you are meant to be, and also frees others in your life to be who they truly are. Whenever you feel a negative emotion, allow yourself to feel it, learn from it and then let it go. If you stop the negative emotion from emerging or continue to hold onto it by refusing to forgive and let go, you keep your focus on the painful experiences in your past, which stop you from moving forward in life. Instead you end up creating the same patterns and experiences over and over again. The characters in the drama may change, but the same lessons keep being repeated. This cycle continues until the moment you decide to look at what the lessons are for you in each and every situation in your life. Once you get what is there for you to learn, you realise that what you thought caused you to feel a negative emotion was a blessing in disguise.

Goal setting

You also need to set some goals. Goal setting helps you become clear about where you are going and what you want. It also helps your unconscious mind know what is required of it.

Your unconscious mind is truly your best friend and it wants to help and please you, but you don't often give it clear instructions. Perhaps you can never make up your mind, so you keep changing direction. Or maybe you have conflicting goals and desires, so you hesitate about making any decisions at all, which is actually a decision in itself. This makes the unconscious mind very confused.

Often you try to rely solely on your conscious mind to find out what you want and how to achieve it, but when you ask the unconscious mind for help, you are much more likely to get the results you desire. The unconscious mind has an enormous amount of information and resources available and is a far greater part of you than you probably realise; it is a very powerful ally and friend.

Watching your thoughts

It is important to remember that the unconscious mind takes everything you think and say very literally, as well as personally, just like a child. This is why you have to watch your thoughts and words. For instance, say you want to advance in your career and have a position

similar to your boss. The only problem is, you think your boss is really tight and greedy, and you find yourself discussing this with your colleagues. Do you think your unconscious mind would want others to say similar things about you when you become a boss? No, of course it doesn't. So instead of helping you achieve your goal, it will sabotage your efforts.

This is why you have to be very clear about what you want and when you see others who have achieved something similar to what you want, you need to tell yourself, "That's what I want!" Always focus on what you want, **never** on what you do not want. Other comments to watch out for are expressions such as, "He really gets on my nerves", "She is such a pain in the neck", "You really give me a headache", or "I'm dying to see you" because the unconscious mind hears you, and since it wants to please you, it will start creating what it thinks you want. This is especially important to remember when speaking to young children. If you say to a child, "You are so naughty", "You are such a bad boy", "You are pathetic", "You make mummy really angry" or "Don't be so stupid" they will believe you. These comments sink into their unconscious minds as beliefs about themselves. It will not be long before the child's unconscious mind starts to act upon these beliefs. I have seen countless children in my practice who have had deeply held limiting beliefs about themselves, such as believing they are stupid, a bad person or a failure. Often these limiting beliefs started as an angry comment by a frustrated adult in their lives, usually a parent or a teacher.

Setting SMART goals

On the positive side, when used in the correct way, knowing that the unconscious mind takes things very literally and wants to be of service, you can use it for goal-setting and easily achieve what you want in life. Set clearly defined and realistic goals using the criteria for a SMART goal:

S – simple
M – measurable and meaningful to you
A – achievable
R – realistic and responsible
T – toward what you want and timed

Look at these guidelines and set goals accordingly. The goal also has to be ecological, meaning it has to improve all other areas of your life and not be at the expense of another area. For instance, if a goal is to advance in your career but this goal also means that you will work long hours, never see your family and not have time and energy for improving your health, then this is not an ecological goal and it will be more difficult for you to achieve it.

In the coaching programme we will go into detail about setting goals for each area of your life, but here I just want you to practice it. So write down several goals you want to have achieved by next week, next month, next six months, next year, next five years and next ten years.

'Perfect Day' exercise

Another good exercise is to write down your perfect day and then your perfect week. How would you be, what would you do, and what would you end up having as a result of this? Then visualise it and see yourself in the picture. Then say to yourself, "I am X, I am doing X, and I have X."

Say, for instance, you want to become a writer and publish books. See yourself writing; visualise your books being published and sold in all the national and international bookstores, bringing happiness, love and joy to millions of people; and say to yourself, "I am a writer", "I am writing books for the highest good of all concerned", and "I now have all my books published." Always make sure your goal is for the highest good for everyone.

Use this knowledge for improving, enhancing and bringing into fruition anything you desire in your life. Everything starts with a thought and a belief that it is possible. Your thoughts are very powerful and creative, so use your mind consciously and constructively. Focus on what you want, and when you know what you want, trace back to see what qualities you will need to have in order to achieve your desired goal. Then be these qualities, do actions from these qualities, and soon this will bring you the manifestation of what you desire. A simple example is someone who wants to have more happiness in life. If he is happy, he will act with happiness, which will then affect others, and they will act with more happiness towards him. What you give you receive. This works with everything in life. Experiment with this and you will soon know from your own experience that this is so.

Finally, after you have set your goals, you need to take action towards achieving them. This means that you need to do everything you can to allow your goal to materialise. If you want to improve in the areas of health, fitness and well-being, then you may need to change the way you eat, start exercising more and have a course of treatments by a qualified complementary practitioner to re-energise your physical vitality. In addition, you may want to release negative emotions, limiting beliefs and decisions to re-balance your mind and meditate daily to re-discover your spiritual self. Then you are well on your way to improving your health, fitness, happiness and well-being.

Focusing on what you want

Whatever you focus on becomes reality in your life. This is because thoughts are creative. Unfortunately, so many people walk around constantly engaging in negative thought patterns, worrying about what might happen. Anthony Robbins writes a beautiful metaphor in one of his books about race-car drivers. They all know that whatever they focus their gaze on, their body (which is part of their unconscious mind) will automatically steer towards. So if they are about to crash into a wall, they keep their focus on the road they want to stay on, **not on the wall**. He also writes about the secret of highly successful people: when they are faced with a problem, they spend 10% of their energy focusing on the problem and 90% of their energy focusing on the solution. So focus on what you want, and you will automatically stay on that path, finding the solutions to any tests you may encounter on the way.

What to do if you are not experiencing well-being

First, you need to find out how you can open the gate to your inner place where you can heal in the most efficient way. We are all different and therefore what may suit one may not suit another. Often you have to try a few avenues until you find what seems best for you. Second, you need to discover the root cause of the imbalance.

Some think that this lies within their physical structure and it is obviously a good place to start. But if you only focus on this aspect of your being you may miss the original cause. I believe the original cause often stems from repressed negative emotions, deeply held limiting beliefs, and imperfect thought patterns. However, at times the cause can be purely physical, such as when you hurt your neck from carrying a heavy load…or environmental, like contracting an illness due to toxins, pollution or radiation. At other times the true cause may be spiritual. Perhaps there is something your spirit wants you to pay attention to or learn from by having this imbalance in your life.

In this book you will start with balancing your mind, because when you release old negative emotions, limiting beliefs and decisions—which are held in your mind—you immediately help your body and your spiritual self to achieve and maintain balance and well-being. So it is to your advantage to do all the meditation exercises outlined in the coaching programme. If possible, find a partner to do them with, and make sure you both have read the relevant chapter thoroughly and fully understand the exercises before you do them. At the end of the programme you will be amazed how much you have changed, and how much more joyful, aligned and energised you feel. This will dramatically and positively change your whole inner perception of your life, which will then be reflected back to you by the positive changes happening in your outer life.

Part II

The Mind

chapter 2

Re-balancing the Mind

The greatest source of stress is not coming from your external world, but from your internal reality—your thoughts and feelings. The effects of emotional and mental stress have long been documented and science agrees that this type of stress is a major contributor to today's illnesses. I believe it is the main cause of physical imbalance.

I also believe that the body reacts to our thoughts and feelings. For instance, if you tell yourself "I feel sad," your posture will reflect that. When you feel sad you tend to slouch, lower your head, avoid eye contact and basically tell the world you are closing off from any contact. Instead, if you tell yourself "I feel really happy," you will adopt an entirely different posture. When you feel happy you tend to walk with more energy, stand up straight, look directly at people in your environment and have a physical expression of being open and receptive to the external world. So in a very basic way you can see how your internal thoughts can affect your physiology, including your breathing and posture. What many people do not realise is that this has an affect on the central nervous system, which determines your hormone output and is directly linked to your emotions. Imagine what happens to your physical and mental well-being when certain thought patterns are being constantly repeated.

Your body is a mirror

The body is run by the unconscious mind which communicates with both your conscious mind and your Spiritual Self, constantly sending you messages about your inner world (your thoughts and feelings) in order to help you maintain balance and well-being in your life. Sometimes these messages come in the form of physical symptoms: your body literally translates what you are thinking or feeling into a physical symptom, although often there is a time delay between when the thoughts occur and when the first symptoms appear.

For instance, if you feel you always have to do everything yourself; that all the responsibility is weighing heavily on your shoulders—is it any wonder if your body eventually reacts with neck and shoulder pain? Perhaps there is someone in your life you would like more control over (such as a parent over a teenager), but you feel the control is slipping through your fingers—then your joints may suffer as a result, especially in your hands and fingers. Maybe someone is being a real pain in the neck and you keep saying to yourself, "He is such a pain in the neck." It is likely your body will hear this and literally produce a neck pain. The body merely acts as a mirror for what is happening within your mind and soul; I have seen countless examples of that in my practice.

Case studies

One such perfect example is Ann, who came to see me for well-being coaching. She had problems conceiving naturally. Her first in vitro fertilisation treatment had been successful and she had given birth to a lovely baby girl. Soon after, she wanted to implant the rest of her healthy embryos; on both occasions she became pregnant but suffered a miscarriage.

Eighteen months before she came to see me, she found out there was nothing wrong with her fertility—and never had been—and that she should be able to conceive and give birth naturally. During our session, Ann remembered how, as a young child, she used to pick little bits of dirt from her navel, and how she used to believe these bits of dirt were actually little babies. She couldn't stop herself from picking them out, and each time she did it, she believed she was killing these unborn babies. This caused her to feel she was a horrible person and was not deserving of having children later on in life. There is little wonder her body did not allow her to become pregnant naturally.

A second example is Julia, a 71-year-old woman, who came to see me for cranial osteopathy. She suffered from upper neck pain, had a feeling of having a sharp lump in her throat, and felt she could not use her voice properly. She had been for numerous tests and they could not find anything wrong with her. During the examination, I felt her upper neck was so tense it actually felt as if she was being strangled. I said this to her and she looked really shocked. Julia then revealed that her ex-husband used to beat her and tried to strangle her at times. A few days after the treatment, Julia phoned and said that the horrible feeling in her throat had gone away, and that her voice was better. At her second treatment she told me that for the first time in 71 years she had been able

to say 'no,' and to verbalise what she actually wanted. She said, "I think it is about time for me to do what I want to do with my life." This is a clear example of how a repressed incident was causing a physical symptom and restricting behaviour. The physical symptom started to clear as soon as the repressed memories were acknowledged and dealt with.

A third example is Sasha, a woman in her early thirties, who came to see me for a breakthrough session. She was happily married with a young child. Sasha suffered from nightmares and anxiety relating to her fear of not being loved and accepted by her husband and child. She feared that somehow they would throw her out, or not want to have anything to do with her. Sasha's medical history revealed she had suffered from four bouts of pericarditis (inflammation of the sac around the heart), and that she was prone to develop a high fever every time she had to do something where she would be noticed.

She came from a troubled family background where she had been abused physically, emotionally, and mentally by her alcoholic father. Whatever she did he would find fault with, which, to him, justified his rage. During her childhood, the abuse was mainly directed at Sasha, although occasionally her mother would be the target. Her younger sibling was usually spared. Sasha started to rebel against her father's behaviour when she was 12, which caused her to be perceived as the troublemaker in the family. None of the others wanted to look at the real issue, instead they preferred to see her as the one causing the problem.

This impossible situation left Sasha with only one choice—she had to remove herself from the family dynamics. She started to find ways of not having to be around her father and eventually moved abroad where she was living when she came to see me.

During our session, she realised that the inflammation around her heart was her body's response to the heartache she had felt growing up. She had never felt her family loved and accepted her for who she was, and the sadness from that had started to restrict her ability to give and receive love; the sac around her heart symbolically restricted the function of the heart. The high temperatures she developed from being noticed was a response to the fear she used to feel whenever her father noticed her, since that was likely to lead to abuse.

She was aware of how different her life was now, with a husband who truly loved and accepted her and a child who felt her mummy was the best person on the planet. She realised she was loved and accepted by them for who she was and that she truly was part of her new family. Since our break-through session some years ago, Sasha never suffered from pericarditis or a high temperature again. She has managed to forgive her father for everything, allowing her to see him for who he is now, rather than who he was in the past. This has freed Sasha to live her own life without the ghosts of feeling unlovable and unacceptable restricting her ability to love and be loved. It is amazing how the body and the mind work!

Emotional and mental well-being

I feel it is necessary to talk about emotional and mental health together, because they are intricately linked. To make it easier, I am going to make a distinction between the two as the **unconscious mind** (the emotional, feeling, intuitive, gut-reacting part of us) and the **conscious mind** (the mental, reasoning, logical, thinking part of us).

The unconscious mind

When you are born you have an unconscious mind. Somewhere around the age of five, six or seven you start to develop a conscious mind. Up to that age you are a little unconscious mind absorbing everything from your environment without any filtering protection. This is why so much damage can be done during early childhood to your emotional and mental well-being. This can affect you for the rest of your life unless you do something about it.

The unconscious mind runs your body and has a blueprint of you in perfect health as well as your current health. It wants to preserve your body at any given moment in time; it protects you from danger, which is why you instinctively know if you are in danger before you actually see it with your eyes. The unconscious mind is the domain of all your emotions and stores all your memories. It will also repress memories and emotions, which you are not able to deal with at the time, in order to protect you. At some point later in your life your unconscious mind may present these repressed memories and emotions to your conscious mind, so the conscious mind can make sense of them and release them.

When you do not deal with the repressed memories and release them, your unconscious mind lovingly draws situations to you, which mirror the content of these repressed memories and emotions, so that you get another chance to deal with them and release them – and heal.

This is why some children who have experienced parental abuse are attracted to partners who may abuse them, or they may even become abusers themselves, when they grow up. Other children who have had similar experiences may have dealt with them and released them so their unconscious minds do not have to draw these experiences to them again. It can also be that some children do not release the wounds from their childhood, and still they do not attract abusive relationships to themselves—instead they may attract a partner who is the complete opposite to their abusive parent. But the repressed emotions have to go somewhere, so they may become angry, depressed or lack energy. Keeping memories and emotions repressed demands a great deal of energy, which is why people feel so much better and lighter when they release them.

You all have repressed memories and emotions. You all have wounds from your childhood. You all have made limiting decisions about yourselves, which restrict the way you function and lead your lives, and you all have been presented by your unconscious minds with the content of these repressed memories. The question is, how do you deal with it? Do you accept the opportunity, learn from it, release it and move on, feeling better and lighter? Or do you desperately stop it from emerging by keeping your conscious mind so busy it cannot possibly acknowledge what is emerging? Perhaps you wallow in it for days, weeks, months or years feeling sorry for yourself and in this way effectively stop yourself from getting on with your life? Or maybe you choose to get angry with people around you, so that you don't have to feel your own inner sadness, fear and/or guilt?

The conscious mind

If your conscious mind—which most of you would equate with being the thinking part of yourself—accepts that you are responsible for your own health, well-being, and everything that happens in your life, then it will deal with the emotions as they come up. It will look for the causes why you feel a certain way, or have discomfort somewhere, and it will seek out the appropriate tools to help you get better again.

By realising you are at cause, you empower yourself to take charge of the situation.

However, if the conscious mind is terrified about what the unconscious mind is trying to present it with, it will stop it from emerging, leaving you feeling exhausted and drained. This can severely affect your health as repressed emotions of anger, sadness, fear and guilt have been linked to various illnesses.

Also, if the conscious mind does not want to take responsibility, it will blame circumstances and other people for the way you feel and for your problems. This can be a huge pay-off and the reason why someone does not want to get better. It may be that the secondary gain of having the problem is greater than actually getting well. Perhaps by being angry the person always gets his own way, because the people he surrounds himself with would rather give in than have an argument. Or someone who has been depressed for a long time due to an unhappy childhood may find it easier to keep being depressed, because in this way she can keep blaming her parents for her unhappiness, which effectively stops her from taking responsibility for her own well-being in the present. It may also be that someone who is ill does not want to get better, because by being ill their family has to do everything for them. If this sounds like you, then please ask yourself if any of these behaviours make you truly happy. There is always a reason why you do things and once you find the reason, you can do something about it and get the results you want.

How to improve emotional and mental well-being

Would you like more happiness and balance in your life? Are you willing to make changes to achieve that? Are you ready to take responsibility for your own emotional and mental well-being? If you answer yes to these questions, then you will undoubtedly benefit from the following suggestions:

• Take time out for yourself. You can only give to others that which you first have given to yourself. So value yourself and your time. Learn to be your own best friend, and to love your own company.

• When you feel emotional or mental discomfort or pain, look at it. Then deal with it and release it. Remember that what you resist persists, and what you look at disappears.

• Regularly spend time with people you love.

• Learn the art of laughing, both at yourself and at life in general. There is no better medicine than laughter.

• Cultivate a habit of always seeing the positive in every situation. There is a positive lesson for you to be found in every encounter and experience you have ever had and will ever have. Once you get the lesson, the negative emotions associated with that event will be released and you will be left with love and compassion.

• Yoga and Tai Chi are examples of physical exercises which are highly beneficial. Incorporate one into your daily routine.

• Writing in a journal is a powerful way of getting in contact with your unconscious mind, releasing repressed emotions and memories, and becoming clear on what you want.

• Visualisation is an effective tool for creating change within the body-mind framework. It gives clear signals to the unconscious mind of what is wanted from it, and also of what is possible. Athletes have used this for many years since it has been found that the body performs far better after you have visualised yourself completing a task successfully. This can be used in all areas of your life, such as your education, career, relationships, health and fitness.

• Breathing exercises can quickly change your emotional and mental state. Rapid, deep breathing will increase your energy and heighten your awareness, while rhythmic, regular, slow breathing will calm your emotions and thoughts.

• One of the most effective ways of balancing your emotional and mental states is through daily meditation. Many people think that meditation is difficult. Nothing could be further from the truth. It is being in that place within yourself where you feel connected with your spiritual self, which allows you to experience perfect well-being. How you get there is up to you. There are many meditation practices and you can find what suits you. Below is a description of an easy and effective meditation.

Meditation exercise to improve emotional and mental well-being

Sit comfortably with your back erect and your feet on the floor. Just relax and close your eyes and breathe in through your nose and out through your mouth in a ratio of 1:1. For instance, breathing in to a count of four and breathing out to a count of four. The breathing should be relaxed and easy.

After a while you may start to breathe normally. That is fine. Just stay within yourself in this space and allow yourself to just be. When thoughts start to interfere, gently send them away.

Now visualise yourself drawing an energizing, red light up through the soles of your feet and into every cell of your body. Feel how this red light completely fills and re-energises your body. Then visualise yourself drawing a peaceful, white light down through the top of your head.

Feel it flow down your spine and into the rest of your body. Feel how this white light fills you with peace and totally re-balances your mind.

Then bring your awareness to the place between your eyebrows. As you remain there, you may notice a blue-white light. When you do, just follow this light. Allow yourself to be surrounded by it, to fully experience it. This is the spark of your spiritual self, or your wise self if you prefer. You will soon start to experience a deep, inner sense of peace and joy. This is the peace and joy from your spiritual self, which now has a chance to flow to your mind and body. From this space within you, you may want to visualise yourself being strong, confident, happy, filled with enthusiasm and energy (or any other positive qualities you want to increase in yourself). You may take the time to talk to your spiritual self. Ask any questions you have and wait for the answers. They may come as words, images or feelings. Thank yourself and life for all that you have and for all that you give to others.

Complementary therapies for re-balancing the mind

Hypnotherapy is an excellent therapy for achieving improved harmony, balance and integration between the conscious and unconscious mind. Here the conscious mind has to start listening to what the unconscious mind is trying to communicate, and unwanted patterns and behaviours—which are always run by the unconscious mind—can be exchanged with more appropriate ones.

Imagery and guided visualisations are powerful techniques for helping you connect with your deep emotions and thought patterns, as well as helping you in assisting them to change.

Neuro-Linguistic-Programming (NLP) is a highly effective method for improving the communication between the unconscious and conscious minds. It has several excellent tools for changing unwanted states and behaviours as well as becoming more aware of what is stopping you from living the life you want to live.

Life and well-being coaching often use a combination of NLP and hypnotherapy and are great when you need help finding balance in your life or defining the steps you need to take in order to get where you want to be.

Timeline therapy® is a relatively new method designed by Dr. Tad James and is a form of hypnotherapy. It is a safe, gentle and highly effective method for releasing unwanted emotions, such as anger, sadness, fear and guilt, as well as releasing limiting beliefs and decisions, such as "I'm a bad person", "I can never make enough money" or "I am unlovable."

Spiritual healing, Huna healing, Reiki and chakra healing are very powerful therapies for helping you to connect with your inner well-being. That is partly because the healer holds a vision of you in perfect health, and as she works on you to bring you closer to that vision, your physical, emotional and mental bodies are able to let go of everything that is blocking you from totally being the highest expression of yourself.

Tibetan medicine and ayurvedic medicine are profound, ancient, spiritual and physical healing systems that can greatly enable the mind to come into balance.

Other therapies known to improve our emotional and mental well-being are cranial osteopathy, Chinese medicine and acupuncture, Rolfing, Reichian therapy, kinesiology, aromatherapy, Bowen technique, homeopathy, and certain herbs and flower remedies.

Learn more about these and other therapies in Part VII.

chapter 3

Coaching Programme for Re-balancing the Mind

Step 1: Values for relationships, family, work and career

The areas that tend to be most involved in our emotional and mental health are relationships, family, work and career. If you did not write down your values for these areas before, now is the time to do so. What is important to you about family? Write down at least ten values. Rank them from 1 to 10 in order of importance. Then ask yourself, "Why is value X important to me?" Write that down also. When you look at what is important to you about family, you may find that some of your values do not support you in experiencing happiness within a family unit. Perhaps one of your values was 'a sense of belonging' and when you asked, "Why is that important to me?" you may have answered, "Because I never felt a sense of belonging within my family as a child," which indicates that you have an 'away from' value (your internal representation of your value is a picture of you having a feeling of never belonging as a child, and you are 'moving away' from that).

Then select a percentage from 1 to 100 that represents how much that is an 'away from' value for you. You may say it is 95% away and 5% towards. This now gives you a clear indication that you have some issues relating to your family values. Ask yourself "What is the underlying, limiting belief which has caused this 'away from' value?" Perhaps the limiting belief is, 'I am unacceptable as I am.' Do this for every value you listed and write down all your underlying limiting beliefs. Do the same with your values for relationships, work and career.

Step 2: Releasing negative emotions

This is a very important step in order to achieve balance of the mind. Holding on to any of these negative emotions will create tension, unhappiness and even illness within your body and your life. For most people it takes less than ten minutes to release a negative emotion. This is because the unconscious mind works and learns very quickly. It only takes longer if you allow the conscious mind to halt the process by trying to make sense of it. It may be useful to do this meditation exercise with a partner who can read it to you, or alternatively you can record it on a tape and play it back to yourself when you want to release a negative emotion. If you have suffered severe emotional pain in the past, or if you go into a deep trance very easily, then find a well-being coach, NLP practitioner or hypnotherapist who can help and assist you in releasing these emotions.

Meditation exercise for releasing negative emotions

Always release the negative emotions of anger, sadness, fear, and guilt in this order. This is because anger and fear are energising emotions (they increase the sympathetic tone), so when you release them you will feel really flat and drained. Allow at least one hour for this exercise. After the four major emotions are released, then you can release other emotions, such as hurt, loneliness, and depression.

Sit comfortably. Allow yourself to completely sink into the stillness within you. Ask your unconscious mind if it is totally willing to assist and support you in releasing this negative emotion here and now. When you get a sense of 'yes', go ahead (if you read this out to someone, get them to nod the head when they get a 'yes').

Now see in front of you a magical, flying carpet that can take you anywhere you need to go in your past, and it can do so at great speed. Step on board this magical carpet. I would now like to ask your unconscious mind:

When was the very first time you felt this _____ (specific negative emotion), the original event, which when released, will cause all the _____ (specific negative emotion) to disappear? If you were to know, was it before, during or after you were born into this life? (wait for an answer)
(If after, ask): If you were to know, how old were you?
(If before, ask): Was it in the womb or before that?

(If in the womb, ask): If you were to know, how many weeks or months of age were you?
(If before, ask): Was it at the time of conception, in a past life or did you inherit it from your parents?
(If in a past life ask): If you were to know, how many lifetimes ago?
(If from the parents ask): From which side and how many generations ago?

Once you get an answer (It will always be before the age of 7. If it is not, then it is not the first event.), say the following:

Now instruct the magical, flying carpet to take you there. Feel yourself lifting up in the air, and travel back into the past, right down inside the first event where you felt this _____ (negative emotion). Notice what is happening in this event and also note if you are aware of the _____ (negative emotion) that is there, too. As soon as you feel the _____ (negative emotion), fly up from this event and go just before the event, so that you look down on what is happening.

If there are other people with you at the event, take the opportunity to speak to each of them from the wise part of yourself. Tell them everything you need to tell them. Let it all out. Then allow them to reply from their wise selves, so they also get to say everything they need to say to you.

Ask your unconscious mind what the positive insights and lessons are for you from this event. These positive insights and lessons have been waiting for you all this time, and they will allow you to let go of your _____ (specific negative emotion) easily. Make sure you get these positive insights and lessons.

Search within your heart to see if you now are ready to say to the other people in this event that you forgive them, or if there is anything else you need to say first before you can forgive them fully. Go ahead and do that now. Then allow them to do the same to you.

(To the practitioner: if original event was during this lifetime say): Reassure the younger you that he/she will never have to experience this again, because you are here now to protect him/her. Then take the younger you inside your own heart and allow him/her to grow up into the wise person you are today.

(To the practitioner: if original event was in a past life or inherited from one of the parents say): Now thank the others involved in this event for doing this work with you.

See a little fire burning at the site of the event. Place your old _____ (negative emotion) in this fire and watch the white-blue heat transform it into a positive emotion. This positive emotion is a gift to you that will help and support you in your journey through life. What is this positive emotion? (give time to answer). Breathe in this _____ (named positive emotion). Let it fill your lungs and as you breathe out, let this _____ (positive emotion) flow to every cell of your being—body, mind and spirit. Do this one more time, please.

Now fly down inside the event again and see how differently you feel about it now that you are enriched with your new wisdom and positive emotions. Notice that all the old _____ (specific negative emotion) is completely gone.

(To the practitioner: if it has not, have the person ask what other positive insights and lessons there are in order to release the emotion fully. If it still does not release, ask if the person is at the first event. If not, have the person instruct the magical carpet to go there now.)

With the _____ (specific negative emotion) fully released, feel yourself travel back to the present time, releasing all the _____ (specific negative emotion) on all the events. Look for the positive lessons in each event and let go of the _____ (specific negative emotion), all the way back to the present time. By doing this you free yourself from the past, so that you can live fully in the now.

When you reach the present time, see a little fire burning there. Place all your old _____ (negative emotion) on the fire, and see how the fire purifies and transforms it into a new, positive emotion. This new, positive emotion is another gift to you, which will allow you to totally let go of all the _____ (specific negative emotion) from your past. Notice what this positive emotion is (give time to answer). Breathe in this _____ (new positive emotion), let it fill your lungs fully, and as you breathe out, let this _____ (positive emotion) flow to every cell of your being—body, mind and spirit.

Now travel out into the future and see how much your future has changed. Notice how you feel so much lighter and happier. Then fly back to the present time. Step off the magical carpet and thank yourself for doing this journey. Then thank life for everything it has already given you. Rest in this peacefulness for a few moments and when you are ready, open your eyes.

Case study

Lucy was a lovely lady in her mid-thirties who had suffered panic attacks for the past 10 years. The attacks always happened on weekends or during school holidays, and would be triggered by anyone (even the dog) who put any demands on her. In addition, Lucy felt she could not allow herself to be happy. As a child, Lucy had been extremely happy but she felt guilty about it because her mother suffered from severe depression. Lucy also felt that she could not voice her needs because she felt guilty about burdening her mother.

When she released anger, sadness, fear and guilt, she realised that all of these negative emotions had been formed during her time in the womb and as a tiny baby, because she had felt responsible for her mother's unhappiness. Lucy realised that her mother's depression was not her fault, and that it was okay for her to feel happy. She also realised that it was now perfectly safe to state her needs. Lucy released a few limiting beliefs and worked out some important goals for herself. Since our session she has been completely free from her panic attacks, is much happier, and feels she can take anything in her stride.

Letter writing combined with meditation for releasing negative emotions

Some people need to have a trained hypnotherapist, NLP practitioner or well-being coach guide them when they do the meditation above. If you are not a trained professional, then the following exercise is very useful because it allows you to release emotions safely and easily by yourself so that you can do it anytime, anywhere.

Take the time now to write four letters (or more, depending on how many emotions you need to release). First, write a letter expressing everything you feel angry about. Let it all out. Then do the same with sadness, fear and guilt. Start each letter with "Everything I feel _____ (specific negative emotion) about." If needed, write about other negative emotions, such as depression, bitterness, loneliness or hurt.

After you have done this, I want you to carefully burn each letter. The fire will purify all the negative emotions contained in the letters.

Then go within and visualise a little fire in front of you. Place all your old anger in this fire. See how the fire purifies it. From the fire a new, positive emotion and a positive insight are slowly rising. This new positive emotion and positive insight are gifts to you, which will allow you to let go of your anger easily and effortlessly. Notice what they are. Then breathe them in. Let them fill your lungs fully. As you breathe out let this positive emotion and positive insight flow to every cell of your being—body, mind and spirit.

Now do the same with the other negative emotions. For each old emotion that is being purified by the fire, a new positive emotion and positive insight will be given to you as gifts. Then with these new positive emotions and positive insights inside every cell of your being, see how your future has changed. Notice how positive, happy and empowered you feel. Know that all the work you have just done has totally changed you, and as you have changed on the inside, your outer life will start to reflect this positive change as well. Keep this feeling and knowledge within you and when you are ready, open your eyes.

Now write a new letter, a thank you letter, for everything you have in your life that is bringing you happiness, love and joy.

Step 3: Releasing limiting beliefs and decisions

This is a very important exercise. Look at your values for relationships, family, work and career. What underlying, limiting beliefs have you made to form your 'away from' values? Start with the limiting belief that has the biggest intensity for you and do the following meditation exercise. It may be useful to do this exercise with a partner or record it on tape so that you can play it back to yourself.

Meditation exercise for releasing limiting beliefs and decisions

Sit comfortably. Close your eyes and focus on your breathing. Go very deep within to that still, inner place where you feel completely peaceful and safe. Identify one limiting belief that you want to release.

I would now like to ask your unconscious mind if it is totally willing to assist and support you in releasing this limiting belief. Go ahead with the exercise if you get an inner sense of 'yes' (give time to answer).

Now see in front of you a magical, flying carpet which can take you anywhere you need to go—anywhere in your past—and it can do so at great speed. Step on board this carpet now and ask your unconscious mind: When was the first time you formed this limiting belief? If you were to know, was it before, during or after you were born into this life? (Wait until you get an answer).

(If it was after birth ask): If you were to know, how old were you?
(If it was before birth ask): Was it in the womb or before that?
(If in the womb ask): If you were to know, how many weeks or months of age were you?
(If before ask): Was it at the time of conception, in a past life, or did you inherit it from your parents?
(If past life ask): If you were to know, how may life times ago?
(If from your parents ask): From which side and how many generations ago?

(Once you get an answer, say): Instruct the flying carpet to take you to this event now. Feel yourself lifting up in the air, and travel back into the past, right down inside the event where you first formed this limiting belief.

See what is happening in this event and notice what it was that caused you to create this limiting belief.

Now fly up from this event and go just before it, so that you look down on what is happening.

If there are other people with you at the event, take this opportunity to speak to each of them from the wise part of yourself. Tell them everything you need to tell them. Let it all out. Then allow them to reply from their wise selves, so they get to say what they need to say to you, too.

Now ask your unconscious mind to give you the positive messages from this event. These positive messages have been waiting for you all this time. Once you have learnt them you can let go of your limiting belief easily and happily. Make sure you get these messages. Also ask your unconscious mind what the highest purpose was for you in creating this limiting belief in the first place.

Search within your heart to see if you are ready to say to the other people in this event that you forgive them, or if there is anything else you need to say before you can forgive them fully. Go ahead and do that now. Then allow them to do the same to you.

(To the practitioner: if original event was during this lifetime say): Reassure the younger you that he/she will never have to experience this again, because you are here now to protect him/her. Then take the younger you inside your own heart and allow him/her to grow up into the wise person you are today.

(To the practitioner: if original event was in a past life or inherited from one of the parents say): Now thank the others involved in this event for doing this work with you.

Now see a little fire burning at the site of the event. Place your old limiting belief on this fire and see how the white-blue heat transforms it into a new, positive and enriching belief. Notice what this new belief is (give time to answer). Then breathe in this _____ (new positive belief). Let it fill your lungs fully, and as you breathe out let this _____ (new positive belief) flow to every cell of your being—body, mind and spirit. Do this one more time.

Now travel back to the present time on the magical carpet and see how all the events between the past and the present time re-evaluate themselves when you are enriched with your new, positive belief. Notice how differently you perceive yourself and your life now.

Then fly out into the future and see how much your future has changed thanks to your new, positive belief. Then fly back to the present time. Step off the carpet and thank yourself for doing this journey. Thank life for everything it has already given you. Rest in this peacefulness for a few moments and when you are ready, open your eyes.

Case study

Roger was a top businessman in his late forties. His wife wanted him to see me, because every time they went away on holiday he ended up working on his laptop instead of spending time with the family. Roger felt that he had a problem with procrastination and it was starting to create problems for him and his colleagues at work; therefore, the need to catch up with work on his holiday. During our session, it became clear that the procrastination was due to three things: 1. It allowed him to have some rest (he worked 16 hours a day, Monday to Friday, and most of the weekends); 2. It manifested itself when he had to do something which really bored him; and 3. It 'bailed him out' from having to face difficult challenges head on.

The first two causes were easy to deal with. He promised his unconscious mind that he would

take regular breaks and that he would delegate the work that really bored him.

He realised the third cause was a limiting decision he had made, so he decided to release it. When he came to do the 'releasing a limiting decision' exercise his unconscious mind communicated with him that the decision was first formed when he was four years old. Roger had hit another little boy in the face, and he was worried that the police would come and take him away (as only a four year old boy can do). Instead of having to face up to what he had done and apologise to the other boy, his father **bailed him out** by taking him to the park to play football. This set up a pattern by which Roger would always bail himself out from having to deal with difficult tasks.

After our session, he proved that he can successfully work with any challenge. He is learning to delegate and allowing himself time to rest. He effectively cut his working day to 9 hours and he only spends one hour working on the weekend. When he last went on holiday with his family he left his laptop at home. His wife is very happy with the results.

Letter writing combined with meditation for releasing limiting beliefs

If you find it difficult to release a limiting belief as outlined above without using a trained professional, this is another option which you can do by yourself:

Take the time now to write down one limiting belief. Then carefully burn the paper. The fire will purify the negative energy held within this limiting belief.

Go within and visualise a little fire in front of you. Place your limiting belief on the fire. See how the fire purifies and cleanses it. Then from the fire a new, positive belief is slowly rising.

This new, positive belief is a gift to you which will allow you to let go of your old belief easily and effortlessly. Breathe in this new, positive belief. Let it fill your lungs fully. Then as you breathe out let it flow to every cell of your being—body, mind and spirit.

Now go back into the past to at least three events where you used to act with your old belief, and see how differently you perceive the situation now in light of your new, positive belief.

With this new belief inside every cell of your being, see how your future has changed now. Notice how positive and empowered you feel. Know how all the work you have just done has totally changed you, and as you have changed on the inside, your outer life will start to reflect this positive change as well. Keep this feeling and knowledge within you and when you are ready, open your eyes.

Now write a letter to yourself expressing what this new, positive belief will enable you to be, do and have in your life.

Step 4: Forgiveness

When you forgive others, you set yourself and them free. You are then able to truly live in the now and not in the past. You are able to fully feel love and compassion within your heart, and you are also able to really see the other person for who he/she is now, not your own past perception of how you expect this person to be. If you have unresolved issues with anyone, and you feel that it is not safe, possible or constructive to talk to the person directly, then the following exercise is highly beneficial. If you are only going to do one meditation exercise to balance your mind, then this is the one. This exercise is also useful to do with children who are having problems with peers, siblings, teachers or parents.

Meditation exercise for forgiveness

Sit comfortably and breathe calmly for a few minutes. Then visualise that you are in a safe space, somewhere you feel completely relaxed and at peace. See a chair in front of you. Invite a person you need to resolve an issue with to come and sit on this chair, and ask the person if he or she is willing to let you heal your relationship.

If you get a sense that they are, open up the top of your head and let universal love energy flow through your head into your heart and out to the person in the chair. Keep sending the person this healing love until you feel it is complete.

Then tell the person everything you need to say. Let it all out. Allow the person to tell you everything he or she needs to tell you. Continue doing this until you both feel complete and that you can find it in your hearts to forgive each other. Then say to each other that you forgive each other. (To the practitioner: if they find it difficult to forgive, then invite them to access the wisdom within them that knows that the other person acts in the best way he/she knows how to, given his/her resources, knowledge and model of the world.)

Then either cut the cords between you (you can do this with a pair of golden scissors), or just integrate the other person within your own heart. Thank each other for having done this work together.

If you cut the cords, afterwards say good-bye and wish the person well on his/her path in life. When you cut the cords, you cut the projection you have of the other person. This allows both of you to be free from the past so that when you see each other again you are free to start afresh.

Sometimes it is an aspect of yourself that you need to forgive. Invite this part of you to come and sit on the chair and do the same process. At the end, integrate this part within you, so that it once again becomes one with the whole of you.

Other times it may be an aspect of yourself that is debilitating you, such as depression. Do the same process with forgiveness, cut the cords and place all the negative energies held in this aspect of yourself on a little fire. Let the fire cleanse and purify all the negative energies until they are gone. Then see a new, positive emotion or energy rise from the fire that will help you on your journey through life. Breathe in this new, positive emotion or energy, and as you breathe out, let it flow to every cell of your being—body, mind and spirit.

See how your future has changed now thanks to the work you just did. See, feel and hear how different you are now, and how your life becomes so much happier and rewarding as a result.

Case study

Elizabeth was a lovely lady in her sixties who came to see me for a break-through session. She had suffered from depression for over 25 years. She had had a very strict, religious upbringing, where her parents had idolised the priest. What the parents did not know was that this priest was a paeodophile, and he had abused Elizabeth from a very young age. She never told anyone, and neither did any of the other girls he abused until over 10 years later. When the truth finally came out the church did not want to deal with it.

Elizabeth had always felt that somehow she had to be punished for being bad, because as she was growing up she was constantly being told that she was born in sin and that if she was not good she would go to hell.

She experienced her depression as a crushing sensation, which suffocated her and caused her to feel helpless. When she came to the exercise of forgiving and talking to her depression, she said it looked like a giant squid, and all this giant squid wanted to do was to destroy her, to kill her. She felt the squid somehow was connected to the church. She kept sending this squid light and healing love, until she felt she could forgive it. Then she cut the cords that bound the two of them together. After that I asked her to visualise a little fire and place all the negative energies held in this giant squid in the fire, and let the fire purify it, until all the negative energies (and the squid) were gone. She did this, and as the last remaining negative energies were purified she let out a big sigh of relief. Her whole body changed and she looked at least 10 years younger. She was very shaken after this exercise, and then a giggling, little girl emerged, and I could see the carefree girl she had once been. Elizabeth could then start to look forward to the future, something she had not done for a very long time.

Meditation exercise for releasing negative emotions relating to a specific event

There may have been specific events in your life that were highly traumatic that you were not able to deal with at the time. If you want to release this trauma now, do the following meditation exercise. However, if the specific event is too traumatic for you to be able to safely release on your own, find a good well-being coach or hypnotherapist who can assist you.

Sit comfortably and breathe calmly for a few minutes. Visualise yourself being in a safe space, somewhere you feel completely relaxed and at peace. See yourself standing in this space and then bring into your awareness the traumatic event.

See the event in front of you with all the people involved, including yourself. See how old you are. If you are a child, or much younger than you are now, also bring in the present day you into the scene. Allow the younger you to really tell all the others everything he/she needs to say. Let it all out. Then allow the others to reply from their wise selves. Keep doing this until the younger you has fully forgiven all the others, and they have said that they are sorry, too.

Then reassure the younger you that he/she will never have to go through this pain again, because you are here now to help and protect him/her. Take the younger you inside your heart and allow him/her to grow up into the wise person you are today, so that this part of you now becomes complete with the whole of you.

Ask your unconscious mind what the positive insights are from this event. These insights will allow you to let go of all the negative emotions from this event. Make sure you get these insights.

Search within your heart to see if the present day you now is ready to forgive the others as well, or if there is anything else the present day you needs to say first before he/she can fully forgive everyone. (To the practitioner: give them time to say what needs to be said. If they find it difficult to forgive, then invite them to access the wisdom within them that knows that the other person acts in the best way he/she knows how to, given his/her resources, knowledge and model of the world. Instruct them to go ahead and forgive now.)

Access the wisdom within you that knows that the others involved in this event probably did the best they could, given their own resources, knowledge and model of the world. Go ahead and tell them you forgive them now.

Now see a little fire burning at the event and place all the negative emotions on this fire. See how the blue-white heat from the fire cleanses and purifies all the negative emotions until they

are all gone. Then up from the fire a new, positive emotion is rising, which is a gift to you, and will help you on your journey through life. Notice what this positive emotion is (give time to answer). Breathe in this _____ (new, positive emotion). Let it fill your lungs fully, and then as you breathe out let this _____ (positive emotion) flow to every cell of your being—body, mind and spirit.

Thank the others for having done this work with you today. Then either cut the cords between you (you can do this with a pair of golden scissors) or just integrate the other person(s) within your heart.

Now see how your future has changed thanks to the work you have done. See, feel and hear how different you are now, and how your Life is becoming so much happier and rewarding as a result.

Case study

Lauren was a 28-year-old woman who came to see me for severe depression. When she was 12, she had tried to commit suicide by swallowing tablets. Her mother realised what Lauren had done, so she got her to vomit up the tablets and then told her not to be so stupid. She never spoke about it to Lauren again. Lauren decided it was *her right to be miserable* and as soon as she moved away from home her depression started. When we tried to release her anger from the past, there was no way her anger was going to allow itself to go away. Instead we did the forgiveness exercise. This was the first time Lauren had been allowed to really let out all the hurt she had felt all those years ago when she tried to commit suicide. Finally after one and a half hours, she found it in her heart to forgive her mother and she could release all the anger easily and effortlessly. After our session, Lauren felt that it was now *her right to be happy*.

Step 5: Goal setting

Now we come to goal setting relating to your emotional and mental health. Write down your goals and the steps you need to take to get there. Start with writing five goals for this week, five goals for this month, five goals for the next six months, five goals for this year and five goals for the next five years. Goals give the unconscious mind a direction, so that it knows what it is you want. All too often we have conflicting goals that produce conflicting results. Use this process to identify if this is the case for you. Look at your goals closely. Are they in alignment with each other? Do they fulfill the criteria of a SMART goal? If they are, then ask yourself the following questions, "Do you believe you can make this happen?" and "Do you believe this will happen?" When you answer 'yes' to both, then do the following meditation exercise.

Meditation exercise for bringing a goal to life

Sit comfortably. Bring the goal you want to achieve into your awareness. What is the last step that needs to happen in order for you to know you have achieved this goal? When you think of that last step, do you have a picture? Good.

Now step into that picture and make it very real for yourself. Make the colours, the sounds and the feelings in the picture as intense as possible.

Then step out of the picture, so that you see yourself in the picture, as if you are looking at a photograph of yourself. Take the picture between your hands and blow four deep breaths into it. This energises the picture. Then place the picture into a pink bubble and ask your unconscious mind when you want to have achieved this goal (wait for an answer). Then let go of your goal and see it float out into the future to the time that is most appropriate. See how all the events between the successful completion of your goal and the present re-evaluate themselves to support your goal.

Then say to yourself: "I am now _____ (your desired goal). This or something better now manifests for me for the highest good of all concerned." From this moment start acting as if you have already achieved your goal, and your unconscious mind and the universe will materialise your goal for you.

Never, ever say: "I want _____ (your desired goal)" because your unconscious mind will then say, "Okay, I will get that for you," and it will produce the result…the want of something. So instead of saying "I want to be successful" say "I am successful."

When you visualise your goal make sure you see yourself in the picture. That means your body is in the picture as if you are looking at a photograph of yourself. It then tells the unconscious mind that this is what you want and it will go out and make it happen for you. If, instead, you are in the picture looking through your own eyes, the unconscious mind thinks it is happening right now, therefore it has achieved it for you, and it will stop trying to make it happen. The unconscious mind cannot tell the difference between what is actually happening and what is being imagined.

Step 6:
Design your ideal life

Take the time now to write down your ideal life. How would you be? What qualities and feelings would you experience? What would you be doing? How would you bring out your essence into the external world, so that others can experience your unique beauty and light? What would you have in your life? Really think about this and formulate your thoughts on paper, until you have a very clear image in your mind what your ideal life would be like. Then do the following meditation exercise.

Meditation exercise for your ideal life

Sit down comfortably. Close your eyes and go within to that inner place where you feel peaceful and happy. Then see yourself as the person you are in your ideal life. Feel all the qualities you have and see yourself doing the actions all these qualities allow you to do. See, feel, and hear yourself fully living the life you desire. Make it really intense for you. Then step out of the picture so that you see yourself in it. Place it inside a beautiful, pink bubble and send it off into the universe. Tell yourself "This or something better now manifests for me, for the highest good of all concerned."

Step 7:
Solving difficult problems

We all experience a difficult situation from time to time. The question is, how do you deal with it? Do you blame others or do you step back to see your own involvement in the situation? Perhaps the other people involved are quite difficult and they have a lot of negative emotions—such as anger—that they dump on you. Do you accept their anger into your life by allowing yourself to get angry back or are you able to detach yourself from their anger and see it for what it is—a cry for help—which has nothing to do with you? The moment you react to someone else's negativity, you become part of their negative energy, and this is what hurts you. Perhaps the problem is mirroring the content of an unresolved and repressed memory that your unconscious mind is very kindly bringing to your attention. Remember that the solution to every problem is held within the problem itself.

Think of a problem you have. Make it very real and intense for you. Write it down and clarify it further. Then ask yourself the following questions and write down the answers. If you start answering "I don't know," say to yourself "I know you don't know, but if you were to know, I wonder what that might be." By asking a question in this way your conscious mind relaxes enough so that your unconscious mind can deliver the answer. Remember, you do have all the answers within.

• Identify and write down the cause of this problem, what you believe about it (this may give you some of your own limiting beliefs), and how long it has been going on.

• When you think of your problem, which emotions do you feel, and where in your body do you feel them? (You can release these later with the 'release negative emotions held in your body caused by unwanted states and behaviours' exercise).

• Look at the way everyone involved in this problem is reacting to it and see how much negative energy they put into it. Do you believe that the problem can change?

• Describe what happened the very first time you experienced this problem.

• Is there a relationship between that first event and your problem as it is now? What has happened since that first event?

• Is there a relationship between your problem and your childhood, as well as your relationship with your mother, father, siblings, or any other key figure in your life? (Do them all separately).

• Ask your unconscious mind, what is the purpose of having this problem in your life, what was the purpose for creating it, and when did you decide to create it?

• If there is anything your unconscious mind would want you to pay attention to, know, or learn so that if you were to do that, your problem would completely disappear, what would it be?

• What are you pretending not to be aware of by having this problem in your life?

• Look at your problem closely. What are the positive insights for you? Once you get these positive insights you will be able to let go of your problem easily.

• Look at what the possible outcome will be when this negative situation is changed into a positive one and compare that with what would happen in the future if the problem stayed the way it is now.

To find out any secondary gain to your problem, ask yourself the following:

• What is this problem stopping you from doing because it is in your life?

• What is this problem allowing you to do, which you like doing, but which you will not be able to continue doing, once your problem disappears?

• When your problem disappears, there may be something you have to do, which you do not want to do. What is it?

You should by now have a very clear idea of how you created this problem in your life, what negative emotions and limiting beliefs you have associated with it, what your unconscious mind wants you to do so as to allow your problem to disappear, and any secondary gain you may have by allowing the problem to continue in your life. Release all your negative emotions, limiting beliefs, as well as any negative emotions held in your body caused by an unwanted state or behaviour

Now formulate the solution to your problem. What would you like to do instead of your problem? How would you like to deal with the situation? How would you be? What would you do and feel? Write it all down. Get real specific. Then do the following meditation exercise.

Meditation exercise for solving a difficult problem

Bring up the solution to your problem in your mind. Then close your eyes and go within. Find the inner stillness.

Visualise a burning fire in front of you. Place your old problem into the fire, and see the negative energy of the problem becoming purified by the blue-white heat of the fire. Once it is completely purified, see a beautiful, pink bubble rise from the fire.

In this bubble you can see your solution and you see yourself acting it out. Now release this pink bubble to the universe and say to yourself, "This or something better now manifests for me, for the highest good of all concerned." Then say to yourself, "I am X (the solution), I am doing X (the solution), I now have X (the solution)." See how your future has changed as a result of you letting go of this old problem. Rest in the knowledge that the universe is bringing the solution into your life.

Case study

Sarah came to see me because she was very angry with her father. She felt she did not even want to call him 'dad'. His 90th birthday was coming up and it was expected that she would let her children make a speech at his birthday party about what a wonderful man he was. Sarah didn't want them to do this but she was worried if they didn't her mum would be hurt.

After we had done this process, she realised the problem originated when she was 10 years old and she told her dad she no longer wanted to go swimming with him on Sundays. This hurt him greatly and he reacted the only way he knew how—by cutting her out of his life. From that day, Sarah felt she no longer existed for him. So she reacted by cutting him out as well. Instead, she would be extra nice to her mum just to hurt him. She would also fight in her mum's corner, since her mum would not stand up for herself.

Sarah's unconscious mind communicated with her that the solution was really very simple. She needed to let go of the pain and stop continuing the pattern she was currently acting out, by allowing her dad back inside her heart, and by not fighting in her mum's corner. That was her mum's role to do, not Sarah's.

In her solution, Sarah visualised how she was able to walk into a room and greet her dad and actually feel happy to see him. She also visualised how she was able to detach herself from the pattern binding her parents together, so that she allowed her mum to stand up for herself, and how she no longer felt the need to rebel and hurt her dad. Sarah discovered that it was actually up to her children to decide whether they wanted to make a speech or not.

Since Sarah did this work, she has been able to forgive her dad and start caring for him, whilst at the same time be clear about her boundaries.

Part III

The Body

chapter 4

Re-energising the Body

When you are born you have enormous vitality and energy within you. Considering that birth is one of the most stressful events you ever have to experience (it has been estimated the baby produces enough stress hormones to potentially kill an adult), this vitality is undoubtedly needed. As a cranial osteopath, I can feel this amazing potency when I treat young children. When parents bring their stressed baby in for osteopathic treatment (common symptoms are colic, constant crying, not being able to sleep, or feed well), very often the baby responds within the first few sessions. This is because of this inherent vitality. Similarly, a young adult who suffers from a shoulder strain, such as an inflammation of the supraspinatus muscle, will feel acute pain, but the inflammation is usually resolved within a few days. However, when an older person gets a similar injury the pain is less intense, and the inflammation often takes several weeks or even months to resolve. The difference is again due to the inherent healing vitality of the body.

Science now thinks that our bodies are designed to live to be at least 140 years old (even this could be seen as a limiting belief) so most of us undoubtedly age faster than we need to. Statistically we live longer than ever before, but that is not the point, if we still only get halfway to what is actually possible. Furthermore, most people over the age of fifty suffer from one ailment or another, so somewhere along the way we go wrong. But where?

Diet

Think of your body as a highly sophisticated car. Some of you drive sports cars, others drive family cars, some are new, others are old. Some need leaded petrol, others unleaded, and a few need diesel. What would happen if you put petrol in a diesel engine? The car would not perform so well.

So how do you know what type of fuel your car needs? The manual tells you. What about your body…does it come with a manual? Yes, just not a written one, and there are so many different suggestions as to how you should eat that many people find it very confusing. However, your body has an inner manual if you just take the time to listen to its signals. If you notice that whenever you eat steamed vegetables and fresh fruits you have more energy, that is your body saying, "I want more of this!" If you eat a piece of chocolate cake with a cup of coffee and your body responds first with a rush of energy and then 20 minutes later it crashes, that is a sure sign your body did not appreciate that food. Listen to your body and whatever makes you feel more energetic, happy and well (without a crash later), eat more of it.

Remember that we may all be physiologically similar, but we each have unique, individual requirements, so what suits one may not suit another. A good example of that is from my own household. I do not eat meat and have not done so since I was sixteen; however, I do occasionally eat fish. When my husband met me, he changed his diet and lost a lot of weight, which he did not want to do. After a while he felt instinctively that he missed red meat. As soon as he introduced it back into his diet his weight returned to normal. So we each have different physical requirements for our own health.

A common finding during pregnancy is that the expectant woman has cravings. Often these cravings are signals from her own 'inner manual' that something is lacking from her diet. During my last pregnancy I suddenly started craving dark organic chocolate, an excellent source of iron. A few days later my routine blood tests came back, which diagnosed mild anaemia. However, by that time my iron levels had already been raised thanks to my own instincts to eat iron-rich chocolate, and I never needed to take any extra supplementation. Another craving I had during the last trimester was sunflower seeds and olives (both very high in essential fatty acids). I used to eat 500 grams of sunflower seeds and two jars of olives per day! What was the reason for this? I later read in a study that the brain of a pregnant woman shrinks because her fatty acid stores are being depleted by the developing baby. Fortunately my body was signaling this to me and I listened.

There are some basic general rules which most healthy diets adhere to, such as:

• Avoid refined carbohydrates, such as white sugar, white flour and white rice.

• Avoid adding salt to your meals, since there is already too much hidden salt in processed food.

• Avoid colourings, artificial sweeteners, and pesticides

• Avoid drinking alcohol.

• Avoid drinking more than one to two cups of coffee or tea per day. Instead drink plenty of fresh, purified water; still mineral water; and some diluted fruit and vegetable juices.

• Eat wholegrain bread, brown rice, whole grain pasta, and lots of fruits and vegetables. Avoid processed foods.

• Always choose organic and free-range foods, especially fruits, vegetables, eggs, meat, and fatty fish.

• Our bodies also need polyunsaturated fat, so use plenty of olive oil, flax seed oil, and increase your intake of fatty fish (unless it is full of heavy metals), avocados, nuts and seeds.

• Appreciate your food, and eat only when you are hungry and in a relaxed state of mind.

Exercise

Good fuel is obviously a requirement for health. Another requirement is physical activity. Children have a very natural way of exercising. They run around for a while, stop, start again and above all they are having fun. Adults tend to sit most of the time and if they do exercise, they go to the gym a few times a week.

It is much better to do daily, gentle exercise, such as yoga, tai chi and Pilates and to do some cardiovascular activity 2–4 times a week with specific muscle strengthening. This gives the body a chance to gently move the joints and muscles as well as stimulate the circulation and immune system on a daily basis, while improving stamina with adequate rest in between. It is of vital importance to keep using the body appropriately. If you do not use it, it will lose its strength and eventually its function. Unfortunately, many people who exercise do so unwisely. They train their bodies in a way that causes their physical alignment go out of balance, or exaggerates already existing imbalances. This in turn, adds stresses and strains to their bodies, which they eventually have to pay a price for. This is why Pilates and yoga are so popular—they both address this imbalance. When done under appropriate supervision, the affected individual can become aware of the problem and begin to incorporate exercises that combat the misalignment. So exercise as often as you want, as long as you feel happy doing it. Exercise is meant to be fun and enjoyable, not a punishment or a must.

Environment

Other factors that contribute to physical health are found in the environment, such as fresh air, good soil nutrients, and unpolluted water. Being in nature itself is not only vital to our physical health, but also to our emotional and mental well-being. When you feel stressed about something, a walk in the woods can do wonders. Or if you feel sad, sitting on a rock looking out at the sea can miraculously allow your sadness to wash away.

Children especially need the calming influence of nature. Which parent has not seen the transformation from a sensitive, upset or angry child indoors to a happy, delightful and carefree child minutes after going outdoors? Mother Nature truly is a great healer and we all need to be surrounded by her and comforted by her embrace.

Complementary therapies for re-energising the body

If you had a very expensive car wouldn't you look after it? Wouldn't you regularly service it to maintain it in perfect condition, so that you could enjoy it longer? Wouldn't you make sure it was always safe to drive? Of course you would—so how is your body any different? Your body is going to be with you until you leave this physical existence, so wouldn't it be wiser to look after it and have it regularly serviced? Yes! You are so lucky to have so many different tools for helping it to perform better. Osteopathy and chiropractic, for instance, are excellent examples of therapies that always look to improve the neuro-musculo-skeletal balance. When your physical structure is in alignment, everything functions better, not only the muscles and joints, but also the blood circulation, the lymphatic drainage, the immune and nervous systems—all contributing towards improved health of body and mind.

Other excellent treatments for stimulating the body's own healing process are Tibetan, ayurvedic and Chinese medicine and acupuncture, reflexology, shiatzu, massage, aromatherapy and healing. Naturopathy and medical herbalism strive to improve the diet and prescribe various herbs and supplements that will help promote the body's healing capacity. Homeopathy works in a similar way through its remedies. Treat yourself to a tune-up soon! You deserve it.

Learn more about these and other therapies in Part VII.

chapter 5
Coaching Programme for Re-energising the Body

Step 1: Values for health, fitness and living

Write down all your values for health, fitness and living (see Chapter Three, Step 1).

Look at your values. Are they supporting you in your goal of being well, happy and living life to the fullest? What limiting beliefs and decisions have you formed that are causing you to have 'away from' values? Make a list of all of them. Be really honest with yourself. Then ask, "How much do I allow myself to fully live?" Where would you be on a scale from 1 to 10, if 1 was not living at all, and 10 was living your life to the fullest? If you are less than 10, you need to find out what limiting beliefs you have and which are stopping you from living your life fully. Write them down. If any more negative emotions come up in relation to these values, release them as well with the meditation exercise for releasing a negative emotion. Then release all your limiting beliefs with the meditation exercise for releasing a limiting belief (see Chapter Three).

Step 2: Releasing old emotional pain in your body

If you suffer from pain anywhere in your body, now is the time to find out the emotional content of such pain. We are all different, and therefore the emotional content will differ from one person to another. If you seem to be aching everywhere, start doing this exercise with your heart. If you are lacking in energy, do the exercise both for your heart and your central nervous system. If you do not know where any organ or part of the body you wish to heal is situated, research it in a book or online. It is vital that you know exactly where a specific organ is and what it looks like, since it will be easier for you to bring your awareness and your intent there. This will aid you in gaining the information you need in order to assist it in healing.

Meditation exercise for releasing emotional pain in your body

(It may be useful to do this exercise with a partner.) As you sink through the emotions, in the end everyone comes to a place where they feel as if there is nothing more there. That is great, because it means you have reached the bottom of your chain of emotions. As you sink through this layer, you come out the other side, which is always positive. This is because in our essence we are all light, all positive and all love. So embrace that bottom layer and sink through it with gladness, because it brings you home to your inner love and joy.

Sit, or lie down comfortably. Start focusing on your breathing. Just feel the breath coming in and going out. Now bring your awareness to your heart. Feel its power and love for you and for the world. Then bring your awareness to the bottom of your spine, and slowly travel up your spine to your neck, then into the base of your skull, top of your head and finally to the area between your eyebrows. Just stay with your awareness there. This is the gateway to your intuitive self.

Now ask your intuitive self to assist you in the healing of your body. Then travel to the area in need of healing. Really allow yourself to sink into it, to rest there fully. Explore the area. What does it look like? Is there an area that looks or feels different from the rest…perhaps a dark, rugged or restricted area, or an area of less vitality? When you find it, go to this area and just sink into it. There will be an emotion there.

Where have you felt this emotion before? If you were to know, how old were you? Allow yourself to feel and experience this memory again. What are you doing in this memory? Is there anyone there with you? Now sink beneath this to the next layer. What is the next emotion? Allow yourself to really feel it. Check if there is anyone there with you in this memory. Now sink beneath this to the next layer. Do the same process here, and then sink to the next layer. Keep doing this until there are no more layers. Then sink beneath the final layer, the one where you feel there is nothing more there. Just sink through it and you come out at the other side.

This other side is always positive. Often it feels like love, happiness or light.

From here, travel back up to the memory which was most intense for you. Go back to that memory, and meet the people who are there, and who were involved in creating this emotion. Ask them if it is okay with them to let you release this emotional pain here and now. See a chair in front of you. Ask the person you feel is the most involved in this memory to sit on this chair. Open up the top of your head and let universal love energy flow through you into your heart and out to the other person. When you feel this healing is complete, allow yourself to speak to this person from the wise part of you now. Let it all out. When you feel you have completely released all hurt and negative emotions, allow the other person to say to you everything he/she needs to say from his/her wise self. Continue doing this until you both have fully forgiven each other. Then say to each other that you forgive each other.

Now either cut the cords between you (you can do this with a pair of golden scissors), or just integrate the other person within your heart. If you cut the cords, afterwards say good-bye and wish them well on their path in life. When you cut the cords, you cut the projection you have of the other person. This allows both of you to be free from the past, so that when you see each other again you are free to start afresh.

If you need to invite another person involved in this memory to come and sit on the chair and do the same process, then do that now. (To the practitioner, give them time to do this.)

Ask your unconscious mind what the positive wisdom is for you from this event. Make sure you get this wisdom.

Now visualise a little fire and place all the negative emotions on this fire. See how the fire purifies and cleanses the negative emotions, until slowly a new, positive emotion is rising from the fire, which is a gift to you and will help you on your journey through life. Notice what this emotion is (give them time to answer) and then breathe in this _____ (named positive emotion). Let it fill your lungs, and as you breathe out let this _____ (positive emotion) flow to every cell of your being—body, mind and spirit, and especially to the area in your body in need of healing.

When this is done, allow yourself to look around the physical area where you used to feel pain. See how it has changed. Notice how much happier and lighter you feel. Ask if there is anything else in this area you need to learn or know, or if you have learned everything so that it now can continue to heal itself completely. Then ask your body how long it will take for it to heal fully. When you get an answer, instruct it to start the healing straight away. Then bring your awareness to your heart and feel its love for you. Just rest here until you feel ready to open your eyes.

Case study

Lisa was a woman in her mid-thirties. She had pain on the left side of her back, just over the area of her fourth rib. She had limited breathing capacity in both lungs, but especially in her left lung. When she did the meditation exercise she saw her left lung being tight and fibrotic with some adhesions in it attaching to the fourth rib. When she felt the emotion there it was fear, and beneath the fear was sadness. This brought up a memory for her of when she was three years old and she saw her father beat up her mother. When her father saw Lisa, he stopped the beating and left. Lisa's mother was so ashamed that she would not look at her daughter, and Lisa felt it was not okay for her to express her fear and sadness over what she had just witnessed. Instead she held it in her body.

In the meditation, she took the opportunity to tell her parents everything she would have liked to tell them at the time. She really let it all out, until she could forgive them in her heart. They also said to her they were sorry and that they never meant to hurt her in this way. Then Lisa asked her body how long it would take for it to heal her left lung and left fourth rib, and it said three months, so she instructed it to start the healing straight away. She also asked if it needed her to do anything else to help in the healing process, and her body communicated with her that it would really appreciate regular treatments, such as cranial osteopathy and acupuncture. When I caught up with Lisa three months later, she was completely free of the pain in her left upper back, and her lung capacity had improved greatly.

Meditation exercise for releasing emotional pain in the body

This is another meditation for releasing emotions held in the body (or just outside the body), caused by unwanted states and behaviours, as well as physical pain. Say, for example, you have a problem with losing your temper with others. When you ask yourself where in your body you feel this behaviour of losing your temper, you may say you feel it in your neck (or any other specific body part). Then when you travel to the area of your neck and sink into the emotion there, you may notice that the emotion there now is anger (or sadness, fear, guilt or any other negative emotion). Once you know the body area and the emotion held there, you can do the following meditation exercise. If the emotion is outside of you, then you need to find out where it is. Common ones are a feeling of a wall in front of you, or a crushing sensation around you.

Visualise a magical, flying carpet in front of you. Step on board this carpet and ask your unconscious mind: When did you first feel this _____ (specific negative emotion) in your _____ (specific body part)? If you were to know, was it before, during or after you were born into this life?

(If after birth ask): If you were to know, how old were you?

(If before ask): In the womb or before that?

(If in the womb ask): If you were to know, how many weeks or months of age were you?

(If before ask): Was it at the time of conception, in a past life or did you inherit it from your parents?

(If in a past life ask): If you were to know, how many life times ago?

(If from your parents ask): From which side and how many generations ago?

Once you have got an answer, instruct the magical carpet to take you to the very first event where you felt this _____ (specific negative emotion) held in your _____ (specific body part). Feel yourself lifting up and flying way back into the past and right down inside the first event.

When you are at this event, allow yourself to feel the emotion that is there and then fly above the event and go just before it so that you are looking down on the event. Notice what is happening there.

If there are other people with you at the event, take the opportunity to speak to each of them from the wise part of yourself. Tell them everything you need to tell them. Let it all out. Then allow them to reply from their wise selves, so they also get to say everything they need to say to you.

Ask your unconscious mind what the positive understanding is for you from this event. This understanding has been waiting for you all this time and it will allow you to let go of your _____ (specific negative emotion) easily. Make sure you get this understanding.

Search within your heart to see if you are ready to say to the people in this event that you forgive them, or if there is anything else you need to say first before you can forgive them fully. Go ahead and do that now. Then allow them to do the same to you.

(To the practitioner: if original event was during this lifetime say): Reassure the younger you that he/she will never have to experience this again, because you are here now to protect him/her. Then take the younger you inside your own heart and allow him/her to grow up into the wise person you are today.

(To the practitioner: if original event was in a past life or inherited from one of the parents say): Now thank the others involved in this event for doing this work with you.

See a little fire burning down at the event. Place your old negative emotion and behaviour in the fire and see how the fire purifies them until they are transformed into a positive emotion and positive behaviour, which will help you on your journey through life. Notice what this positive emotion and positive behaviour are. (Give time to answer). Breathe in this _____ (named positive emotion) and _____ (named positive behaviour). Let them fill your lungs and then let them flow to every cell of your being—body, mind and spirit. Do that one more time.

Once you have done that, fly back inside the memory, and this time step off the carpet and walk around at the event. Notice how positive and empowered you feel now and see how you perceive the situation so differently. Notice that the negative emotion is gone. That's good.

Now step on board the magical, flying carpet again and travel back to the present time only as quickly as you can allow all the events in your life to re-evaluate themselves thanks to your new positive understanding.

Then travel into the future and allow yourself to notice at least three events in the future where if they were to have happened in the past you would have reacted with your old emotion and old behaviour, but see how you react so differently now.

Then come back to the present time and know how all the work you have just done has totally changed you. As you have changed on the inside, your outer life will start to reflect this positive change as well.

Case study

Alex was an eight-year-old boy, who was brought to see me because he worried constantly, especially on a Sunday night and Monday morning before going to school. He would feel really sick in his stomach when he started to worry. We checked what the emotion was in his stomach and it was sadness. We then started with releasing anger, which he felt the first time when he was one year old and his big sister bit his toe. (When doing this exercise with children be prepared to work quickly, because they release issues very fast. Also, they may prefer pretending to be Superman or Superwoman, flying through Space and Time, instead of stepping on board a magical, flying carpet.) When I asked him when was the first time he felt sadness, he said that it was when he was in his mummy's tummy. So we traveled back there, and he realised he had thought then that his mother did not want him. He also had worried that she would not have time for him, since she already had a child. Alex took the opportunity to tell his mum all of his worries and she then replied that she did love him, and that she really did want him. He immediately let go of the sadness. Since our first session, he stopped worrying before going to school, and he felt that he was 70% better.

At our second session *Alex still felt worried about when he had to enter into new situations where he did not know anyone, because he thought that no one would like him*. He felt this worry in his throat and the feeling there was a bit of sadness, like a lump in his throat. So we went back to the first time he felt this lump. It was while he was in the womb, just before being born. He felt safe in the womb and did not want to be born, because *he worried that he was now entering into a new situation where he did not know anyone, and maybe his family would not like him*.

Alex talked to his whole family and also his brother who was not yet born. This made him realise that they all really loved him. He also learned that slight worry before doing something new can be excitement about starting out on a great adventure, and life is an adventure. He then released fear and guilt, both of which he first felt during birth. The fear was from the actual birth itself because it was so quick. The guilt stemmed from him feeling guilty about taking up so much of his mummy's time, which she then could not spend with his big sister. He learnt that a bit of fear sometimes is normal and okay, and that his mum had enough love and time for both him and his sister. Since the session, Alex has been a much happier little boy, daring to enter into new situations, and his mum is delighted with the results.

Step 3: Goal setting

Write down your goals for your health, fitness and living, and the steps you need to take to get you there. Start with writing five goals for this week, five goals for this month, five goals for the next six months, five goals for this year and five goals for the next five years. Goals give the unconscious mind a direction so that it knows what it is you want. All too often we have conflicting goals that obviously produce conflicting results. So use this process to identify if this is the case for you. Look at your goals closely. Are they in alignment with each other? Do they fulfill the criteria of a SMART goal? If they do, then ask yourself two questions, "Do I believe I can make this happen?" and "Do I believe it will happen?" When you answer 'yes' to both, then go ahead and do the meditation exercise for bringing a goal to life (see Chapter Three, Step 5).

Summary of re-energising the body

If you eat healthfully and lovingly, exercise daily, spend time regularly in nature, have complementary treatments when needed, release old emotional hurts and limiting beliefs, as well as aligning your values and goals to support your physical health and life, then you are well on your way to achieving and maintaining excellent physical health. If, however, you do not care what you eat, never exercise, never bother having any complementary treatments even when your body and mind cry out for it, and never take responsibility for your own health and well-being by releasing negative emotions and limiting beliefs, then you will undoubtedly age much faster than you need to, and you are setting up a fertile ground for 'dis-ease' to develop.

Part IV

The Spiritual Self

chapter 6

Re-discovering the Spiritual Self

Now we come to your spiritual aspect. The words 'spiritual self' may have a different meaning to each of you, but I define it as the part of you that existed before you were born and the part of you that continues after your physical body dies.

Your spiritual self communicates with your unconscious mind, which in turn communicates with your conscious mind. The spiritual self has an endless amount of energy, and is always loving, regardless of what you do. When you have a strong connection with your spiritual self you tend to feel more alive, energetic and whole. Sadly, many people are so disconnected from this part of their being that they don't even know it exists. This has created an enormous split within us. Some don't even know we have an unconscious mind. Imagine what a split that would be...the conscious mind thinking it totally runs the show! I prefer to have the conscious mind, the unconscious mind and the spiritual self all working together: the conscious mind being responsible for goal setting, being aware of anything that stops me from experiencing happiness and well-being, and listening to the intuitive voice of the unconscious mind; the unconscious mind being responsible for realising the goals set by the conscious mind, releasing anything which stops me from experiencing happiness and well-being, and improving the communication between the conscious mind and the spiritual self. The only link between the conscious mind and the spiritual self is through the unconscious mind.

The importance of a spiritual connection

It has long been known that people who are seriously ill tend to survive longer or heal quicker when they believe in a power greater than themselves, such as God, Spirit, the universe or whatever they may call this force. Many people also turn to this part of their being for the first time when they experience extreme emotional pain and turmoil and find that it truly comforts them. I believe this is because our spiritual self has always been there with us and when we allow it to enter into our lives, we feel its power, love and energy transmitted through the physical, mental, and emotional layers of our being. This is the most powerful healing tool of them all. Our spiritual self is so vast—so much more than we can consciously comprehend—that to the spiritual self anything is possible, even miraculous cure of physical illness.

When you are in alignment with your spiritual self, your thoughts and feelings become calmer and more focused. It does not mean everything suddenly is easy in your life, but it does mean you now have access to something greater than your own personality and it takes the strain and burden away from having to do it all by yourself. It is also important to have goals in life, to know where you are going, and head in that direction. Otherwise, you wander around aimlessly only achieving a fraction of what is possible. At the same time, when you are too attached to the outcome—when not achieving some of your goals is not okay for you—then you are not trusting that life brings you everything you need, and ultimately you are not trusting your spiritual self. This blocks your connection that ironically blocks you from achieving your goals. The best way to achieve what you want is by trusting that life is perfect as it is—whatever it may bring you—and choosing to deal with it in a loving, compassionate, appropriate and detached way.

This allows you to 'un-hook' your emotional attachment to having life be a certain way, which frees up an enormous amount of energy, which in turn can be put to better use somewhere else. By being in contact with your spiritual self, it is so much easier to be happy with what you have and what is coming your way, while at the same time looking for ways to improve your life.

Setting boundaries

Being loving and compassionate in the way of the spiritual self does not mean that you allow others to treat you wrongfully. There is a saying that if someone treats you badly, the first time you forgive them, the second time it is shame on them, and the third time it is shame on you for allowing it to continue.

If you are in an abusive relationship, for example, what your spiritual self most likely would want you to do, is forgive the abuser for everything that has happened, forgive yourself for allowing it to happen, set your boundaries, and release the abusive person from your life in a detached, loving and compassionate way. This allows you to take charge of your life and create the life you want. The abuser will either wake up and learn from you setting your boundaries, or find someone else who is willing to play the victim. The only thing you can do is to change yourself, you can never do it for someone else. If you fool yourself into thinking that "if only this person would change, then everything would be fine," then you are giving your power away…you are at effect from your external world and you will never fully achieve balance and happiness in your life. You are also doing a disservice to your abuser, since he or she is allowed to continue with this behaviour, which will effectively stunt his or her growth and happiness.

How to improve your spiritual well-being

Prayers and meditations are common forms of improving your connection with your spiritual self. All religion and spiritual practices advocate this, albeit in different forms. You can immediately feel the benefit from practising these regularly. As your being becomes more peaceful, loving and calm, you allow your mind to stop running around frantically, and come into closer contact with your spiritual self.

One of the most important lessons we all have to learn as human beings is the art of forgiveness. When you are angry with another person, the person you hurt the most is yourself. For every unkind thought, for every harsh word spoken, you cut the wound within you deeper and deeper, which causes you to feel even more unhappiness and anger.

The moment you truly forgive, your anger melts away and the wound heals. You are able to feel and connect with the love within you, which releases you from the bondage of anger, sadness, fear and guilt. As it releases you, the person you forgive is also set free.

The forgiveness has to be unconditional, just like a loving parent forgives a child who throws a tantrum. The wise parent knows the child does not understand why she is acting this way so it is very easy for the parent to continue to love the child, while at the same time—gently and with great tenderness—teach the child what is acceptable and loving behaviour. The wise parent also knows not to place too much expectation on the child, but accept her just as she is. The same applies to adults. We are just bigger versions of children… we still do not know why we act in a certain way. The next time someone is upsetting you, see them as a small, lost child; love them for the magnificent, human being they are; forgive them for their actions; and lovingly and compassionately set your own boundaries.

Remember that perception is projection. This means that you only perceive your reality according to your values and belief systems, which are based on your past experiences. This is why when ten people experience the same scenario they will have ten different accounts of what happened. The next time someone is annoying or even infuriating you, take a good look within yourself to see what it is this person is representing for you. Perhaps it is reminding you of issues you have not dealt with yet and this annoying person is actually bringing you a gift by allowing you to look at it again, learn from it, and release it. Every time you forgive your enemy, you forgive yourself, for what you perceive in him as something wrong, is really your own wound. When you experience difficulties, take heart in knowing that it is really just a lesson being presented, and once you get the positive wisdom, you are able to release yourself from all the pain and move on.

Complementary therapies for spiritual well-being

Life and well-being coaching, break-through sessions using NLP, timeline therapy® and hypnosis are highly effective in restoring well-being within your whole self and balance in your life. Tibetan, ayurvedic and Chinese medicine are profound in restoring balance within the body-mind-spirit framework. Various forms of healing are highly beneficial for balancing your physical, emotional, mental and spiritual bodies. Higher self therapy from the Hawaiian Huna traditions, chakra visualisation and meditation are all helpful for spiritual well-being.

Learn more about these and other therapies in Part VII.

chapter 7
Coaching Programme for Re-discovering the Spiritual Self

Step 1: values for your spirituality and personal development

Now is the time to do your values for your spirituality and personal development (see Chapter Three, Step 1). Look at your values honestly and objectively. Check for any 'away from' values. Write down which limiting beliefs you have. If any negative emotions come up in relation to your values, release them as well with the meditation for releasing a negative emotion (see Chapter Three, Step 2), and then release all your limiting beliefs through the meditation for releasing limiting beliefs (see Chapter Three, Step 3).

Step 2: Forgiveness

We have discussed forgiveness many times throughout this book. If you are only going to do one exercise that will allow you to experience more of your spiritual self, then do the medita-

tion for forgiveness (see Chapter Three, Step 4). This will allow you to live in the now and not in the past.

Step 3: Goal setting

Finally we have goal setting for your spirituality and personal development. Write down your goals for each area and the steps you need to take to get you there. Start with writing five goals for this week, five goals for this month, five goals for the next six months, five goals for this year and five goals for the next five years. Goals give the unconscious mind a direction so that it knows what you want. All too often we have conflicting goals that produce conflicting results. If this is true for you, this process may be very helpful. Look at your goals closely. Are they in alignment with each other? Do they fulfill the criteria of a SMART goal? If they are, ask yourself two questions, "Do I believe I can make this happen?" and "Do I believe it will happen?" When you answer 'yes' to both, do the meditation exercise for bringing a goal to life (see Chapter Three, Step 5).

Step 4:
Connecting with your inner wisdom

Accessing your inner wisdom is something you do frequently, whether you are aware of it or not. Your unconscious mind and spiritual self are in constant communication. Some of you find it easy to hear and interpret these messages; however, all of you have been aware of this inner guidance at one time or another. Have you ever had a gut feeling—a message from your unconscious mind—about something and it turned out to be true? Of course you have. Often what happens is you instinctively feel you should take a particular course of action but your conscious mind talks you out of it. Later you realise you should have listened to your instinct. So pay attention to those tiny little whispers, because your inner wisdom is held within them. The following is a meditation exercise which helps strengthen your connection with the voice from your unconscious mind and spiritual self.

Meditation exercise for connecting with your inner wisdom

First, think of a problem you want to find a solution to. State it as a question that can only have a 'yes' or a 'no' answer. Write the question down.

Sit comfortably. Bring your awareness to your breathing. Just notice your breath going in and going out, in and out. Then place your awareness between your eyebrows until you see a blue-white light shining there. Immerse yourself in this light. In this light you can sense your spiritual self greeting you.

Ask your spiritual self the question and then in your mind's eye see yourself acting out the answer 'yes' to the question. Notice your gut response. How do you feel about taking this course of action? See if your spiritual self has anything to communicate to you about it.

Open your eyes and make your mind go blank. Then close your eyes and find your inner stillness again, before you bring your awareness to the area between your eyebrows. Stay there until you feel and see the blue-white light of your spiritual self.

Then repeat the question again, and this time in your mind's eye, see yourself acting out the answer 'no'. Notice your gut response and allow your spiritual self to communicate its response to you. Then make your mind go blank.

From having listened to your gut response (your unconscious mind) and your spiritual self, you will have a very clear answer to your question. See yourself acting out your desired course of action. Place this image in a pink bubble and release it to the universe, while saying, "This or something better now manifests for me for the highest good of all concerned."

Case study

Marie was a lady in her early forties who came to see me for a break-through session because she was confused as to whether she should stay in her marriage or not. She liked her husband but she did not feel sexually attracted to him. He, on the other hand, loved her more than anything. She had separated from her husband to be with her lover, but did not live with her boyfriend. Everyday she would go home and cook for her husband and spend time with their children and then at bedtime she would go back to her own flat. So which of the two men should she choose? After a long and lengthy session, where her unconscious mind and conscious mind were not co-operating with each other, we finally did the meditation for connecting with your inner wisdom. The solution became very clear for Marie. What her unconscious mind wanted her to realise was that she did love her husband, it was just that she had a limiting belief that it was not okay for her to be sexually attracted to her husband. This limiting belief started when she was 10 years old when she accidentally saw her brother naked. This had so embarrassed her that she made the decision that it was not okay to be sexually attracted to her brother. Her husband was similar to her brother and therefore she had unconsciously made the connection that it was not okay for her to be sexually attracted to him. When she was 12, her brother married a girl who did not want him to have much contact with his mother or sister, because she felt threatened by their close bond. Her brother obeyed his wife's demands, and this hurt Marie so much that she made the decision that the man she married had to love her more than she loved him, so that he would never leave her (like she felt her brother had left her). After having released these two limiting beliefs she was able to go back to her husband and truly give the relationship all her energy and love.

Step 5:
Gratitude

When you focus on things that you can be truly grateful for in your life, the more positive experiences you will receive. This is because whatever you focus on multiplies and it is much easier to give to someone who is appreciative. Have you ever had the experience of giving something to a friend or family member and they were truly thankful? How did you react? Didn't you want to give them even more? Of course you did. And have you ever had the experience of giving to someone and they did not appreciate it? Perhaps they felt it was not good enough or they made some complaints about it? How did

you react? Did you feel that it was no use in giving this person anything since they did not appreciate it anyway? The universe is no different from you. If you always complain about what you receive in life and you feel that it is not good enough for you, then don't be surprised when you stop receiving good things, and negative experiences come your way instead.

Gratitude also teaches you to give and receive without expectations. Take the time now to write a Gratitude Letter to yourself about you and your life. Then write a Gratitude Letter to each of the key people in your life, including all your family members (even those who have passed away). Really focus on all their positive qualities and all the gifts of understanding and wisdom they have given you by being in your life. When you do this you will find that even past negative experiences have something positive contained within them.

Step 6:
Re-checking values

This is when we bring it all together. When you have done all the exercises in this book, your whole internal world will have changed, especially your values. When you have released negative emotions, old emotional hurts, limiting beliefs and decisions, then all your 'away from' values will have disappeared and you will be left with all your values being 100% 'toward'. This will have a tremendous impact on your life and the way you relate to it. Take the time to write down the different values you have for each area of your life now (avoid looking at your old values just yet). Start with the values for the area in your life that was not working very well before. What is important to you about this area now? Write down at least 10 values and rank them from 1 to 10 in order of importance.

Then ask yourself why this value is important to you. Check how much this value is a 'toward' value now. When you have done all the exercises in the coaching programme you will be left with all your values being 100% 'toward'. So is yours 100% now? Great! If not, check what is stopping it from being 100% and release that limiting belief or negative emotion with the exercises in this book, until it becomes 100% 'toward'.

Now do the same with the values for all the other areas. Compare these new values with your old values. Notice how much you have changed. And know deep within you that as you have changed your inner world, everything else will change for the positive, too. The outside world is only a reflection of your inner world.

Step 7:
Meditation exercise for healing your inner child and meeting the 'future you'

Finally, it is time for you to fully heal your inner child and meet the 'Future You'.

Go within to that still place, where you feel relaxed and at peace. Then draw in light through the top of your head. Let it flow down your spine and into the rest of your body. This light is filled with love and joy.

Visualise the 'baby you' standing n front of you. Hold this tiny baby in your arms and send it as much love as you possible can. Then tell this lovely baby everything you need to tell him/her. Allow the 'baby you' to do the same back. Then reassure the 'baby you' that you are here now to look after it and love it, and that from now on

he/she is completely safe. Then take this baby inside your heart and allow him/her to grow up into the wise person you are today.

Now see the 'five-to-six-year-old you' standing in front of you. Give this beautiful child a big hug and send him/her as much love as you possibly can. Then tell him/her everything you need to say and allow him/her to do the same back. Then reassure this child that he/she is completely loved and safe now because you are here to look after him/her. Then take this child inside your heart and allow him/her to grow up into the wise person you are today.

Now see the '9-to-10-year-old you' standing in front of you. Send this lovely child as much love as you possibly can. Then tell him/her all that you need to say and allow him/her to do the same back. Then reassure this child that he/she is completely loved and safe now because you are here to look after him/her. Then take this child inside your heart and allow him/her to grow up into the wise person you are today.

Now see the 'teenage you' standing in front of you. Send this teenager as much love as you possibly can. Then tell him/her everything you need to say and allow him/her to do the same back. Then reassure this teenager that he/she is completely loved and safe now, because you are here to look after him/her. Then take this teenager inside your heart and allow him/her to grow up into the wise person you are today.

Now visualise a mountain in front of you. On top of this mountain is the 'future you'. See a path leading up to the top of this mountain. Follow this path and feel yourself becoming lighter and lighter as you ascend the mountain. When you reach the top see the 'future you' coming towards you to greet you. Notice what the 'future you' looks like, and what qualities he/she has. Ask the 'future you' any questions you have, and wait for the answers. They will come, either as words, feelings or images.

Your 'future you' has a message for you. This message is a gift to you, a positive message which will help you on your journey through life. Make sure you get this message. Now feel yourself merge with the 'future you', so that you fully integrate all the knowledge, wisdom, love and compassion your 'future you' has.

Look at the view from this mountain and see how much you and the world you live in have changed as a result of your new understanding, healing and wisdom

Thank the 'future you' and know that you can meet up here on the mountain top any time you wish. Then start the descent down the mountain filled with wisdom, love and joy.

When you feel ready, open your eyes and lovingly embrace your new life to the fullest.

Part V

Bringing It All Together

chapter 8

What To Do Next

What to do if dis-ease has manifested

Stop giving yourself a hard time if you have a so-called 'dis-ease'. Realise it is your body, mind and spirit's way of communicating with you—that they need your attention—that you are not in alignment. This is because your body (and therefore also a 'dis-ease') is part of your unconscious mind, which communicates with both your conscious mind and spiritual self.

A 'dis-ease' is just a healing crisis, the body's (unconscious mind's) own attempt to heal you, to get you back into balance.

It does this because it wants to help you. For what purpose? Well, just imagine for a moment that the universe you live in is made of love. You are love and everything you see around you is love. Love wants you to grow and expand, because it wants you to experience and know love even more. It wants you to become whole in body, mind and spirit, and it senses when you are not completely whole. Love knows of the wounds within you, which are blocking you from experiencing wholeness, and it will send you challenges that mirror the essence of those inner wounds. It does this so that you get a chance to become aware of these wounds, to learn from them, release them and in this way move towards wholeness, happiness and perfect well-being.

Sometimes these challenges come in the form of an awkward relationship, an obstacle in your career or a feeling of being 'stuck'. At other times, these inner wounds have taken on a physical manifestation in your unconscious mind as a 'dis-ease' of the body and/or the mind. So in this way a 'dis-ease' is just love's way of showing you your own blockages, of making you aware of these inner wounds so that you can learn from them and release them.

At any given moment you have a choice of how to react to each challenge. You can choose to react with anger, fear, blame and resentment or you can choose to see it as a positive learning opportunity for healing and growth. When you choose the latter it is easier for you to deal with the challenge in a loving, compassionate and resourceful way. This makes it easier for you to free yourself from the negativities of the past, which enable you to let go of everything that is blocking you from experiencing wholeness and perfect well-being. In this way your unconscious mind is healed, your body, mind and spirit are aligned, and you are able to experience and know love even more.

So look for the fabric of love which is present everywhere in you, in your life, in your relationships and even in a so called 'dis-ease'. Perhaps this 'dis-ease' wants you to take the time to pay attention to something? Maybe it is giving you the chance to heal repressed negative emotions and memories from the past? Or is it bringing you positive experiences by being in your life?

When you allow yourself to see the gifts of love contained within these positive experiences, you abolish the fear associated with 'dis-ease' and death. This has a tremendously beneficial effect on the vitality of your body, which makes it much easier for your body and mind to restore health and well-being.

You are so much more than your genetics

You are all born with different genetic tendencies towards various traits, including illness. This does not mean that you will develop a particular illness, it just means you have a greater tendency to do so. What makes one identical twin develop type 1 diabetes and not the other twin? Only in 40% of identical twins do they both develop the illness. The answer lies in the thoughts, values, beliefs and choices that they each make. So empower yourself with positive and balanced thoughts, change the values and beliefs which do not serve you, and replace them with nurturing ones. Find the positive lesson in any given situation and choose to focus on what you want. Then start taking full responsibility for your own life and well-being. Remember that life only has the meaning that you attach to it.

What to do if you feel discomfort

If you are experiencing physical or emotional pain, seek out the appropriate advice for helping you get back into alignment. Complementary treatments work with the body and the mind to help restore balance, which then allows health

to manifest and 'dis-ease' to loosen its hold. It is important to be under your medical practitioner's care if you have a serious illness; complementary therapies can work alongside your orthodox medical treatment.

This book covers a whole range of conditions and will give you a variety of tools for improving your health, taking charge again and empowering yourself to fully live the life you are meant to live.

Always remember that when you have complementary treatments, it is not the practitioner who is making you better. He or she only facilitates the healing process. It is the physical, emotional, mental and spiritual aspects of you that are making you better. Likewise, it was you that made yourself ill in the first place by holding on to past suffering of negative emotions and old emotional pain, by forming limiting beliefs and decisions about yourself and your life, and by not being able to forgive yourself and others for past mistakes and unconscious actions. In this way you were not being true to your authentic self and you were also not caring about the well-being of your body, mind and spirit. When you fully realise this you truly empower yourself to change your circumstances; your physical, emotional, mental and spiritual well-being; and your life.

If you feel you could benefit from more happiness, peacefulness and health, then follow the guidelines outlined in this book. When needed, see a qualified complementary practitioner, who is passionate about helping you achieve better health. Remember to treat your mind, body and spirit with respect, because they allow you to experience more of life and love. A **re-balanced mind** makes it easier to create a **re-energised body**, which in turn allows you to connect more easily with and **re-discover your spiritual self**. When they are all in alignment, you have found the key that leads to that inner place where perfect well-being for life exists.

Part VI
Conditions

Asthma

This is recurrent spasm of the small muscles of the bronchial tubes and excessive mucus secretion into the lungs, which leads to wheezing, difficulty breathing, tightness in the chest and coughing up mucus. There are two types of asthma—extrinsic and intrinsic. Both types are due to a hypersensitivity, but the first one is more of a true allergy induced reaction (such as pollen and dust mite), whilst the second is more of a bronchial reaction, which can be triggered by exercise, cold, stress, infection and pollutants.

What causes it?

Asthma is very common and the incidence is rising rapidly. This may be due to increased stress on the immune system, such as a lack of breast-feeding, weaning too early, introduction to inappropriate solids, chemical pollution of the environment, genetically modified foods, and food additives.

A difficult birth may sometimes be a predisposing factor for developing asthma. There are several reasons for this. Perhaps the baby did not take a good first breath, thereby not 'kick-starting the spark in the motor' of the body and the lungs properly. Or maybe the birth produced residual tension in the skull, neck, thoracic spine, ribcage and diaphragm preventing the lungs, bronchial tubes and ribcage from functioning optimally.

Other possible causes

• Allergies especially to milk, wheat, eggs, fish, shellfish, nuts, peanuts, chocolate, citrus and food colourings
• Allergens, such as pollen, dust mite and mould
• Food additives
• Birth trauma
• Spinal dysfunctions (cervical and thoracic)
• Suppressive treatments, such as treating colds and bronchitis improperly
• Poor circulation and poor elimination
• Stress and emotional upset
• Exercise that induces asthma
• Cold and dry air
• Respiratory infections
• Smoke
• Low stomach acid
• Hypoglycaemia
• Alcohol abuse and liver toxicity
• Certain medications, such as aspirin, ibuprofen and beta-blockers
• Poor functioning of the gastro-intestinal tract
• Heavy metal toxicity
• Heavy use of chemical cleaning materials in the home

What are the psychosomatic causes?

Asthma, considered within the metaphysical and psychosomatic aspect, often indicates an inability to breathe for oneself due to suppressed emotions, such as anger, fear or sadness, which have been forced to be locked in under strict control, therefore leading to an inability to fully breathe out and let go. Last, but not least, a difficult birth is a very frightening experience for a baby, and it may set up a fear of life itself.

How can I help by changing my diet?

• Increase consumption of vegetables and fruits, except citrus fruits (common allergen).
• Eat plenty of seeds, such as pumpkin, sesame and sunflower.

What should I avoid?

• Eliminate all common food allergens, such as dairy, meat, fish, shellfish, eggs, wheat, sweets, chocolate and refined foods for at least three weeks, and then introduce one food at a time to see which ones are causing an allergic reaction (see **Food Allergies**). In some cases goat yoghurt is allowed.

• Always avoid salt, since excess salt increases sensitivity to histamine. It is also wise to completely eliminate sugar, food additives and piped water, and consume coffee, tea and alcohol very rarely.

What should I supplement my diet with?

• Take one tablespoon of olive oil daily for its fatty acid content. Also take flax seed oil and/or fish oil.

• Raw honey is good for the whole immune system (just be careful if you suffer from pollen allergy).

• Get good nutritional support, such as vitamin A, vitamin C with bioflavonoids, vitamin B-complex (especially B6), magnesium, zinc and selenium. If dairy products are eliminated it may be necessary to supplement with calcium.

• Ginkgo biloba may help to prevent bronchial constriction and liquorice root has an anti-inflammatory action. Onions and garlic are good too.

• Green tea is a good anti-oxidant.

What else can I do to improve my health?

• Drink lots of filtered or bottled spring water to decrease mucus build up.

• Strengthen your immune system to prevent infections.

• Regular hot and cold packs to chest (see **Therapies**). This stimulates circulation to the lungs, bronchial tree, ribcage and muscles, which helps improve their function.

• Avoid extreme, cold weather. Wear a scarf over your face to protect your lungs.

• Avoid smoking or smoky environments of any kind.

• Avoid wall-to-wall carpets. Replace with wooden, tile, or vinyl floors as they are easier to clean and do not attract as much housedust mite.

• Avoid using chemical cleaning products. Clean with natural cleaning products instead.

• Various yoga and Pilates exercises help by improving breathing and by balancing your neuro-musculo-skeletal system. Especially useful are the Spinal Twist, the Cat, the Pelvic Bridge, and slow controlled breathing exercises.

How can I improve my emotional, mental and spiritual health?

It is important to decrease the stress levels in your life. Regular practice of relaxation techniques are recommended, such as meditation, breathing exercises and visualisations. The importance here is to calm the central nervous system, whilst improving breathing ability. Sit or lie with your spine straight and breathe in through your nose and out through your mouth at a ratio of 1:1. For each exhalation feel your muscles relax starting with your feet and slowly work your way up to your head. Then feel the small muscles between your ribs relax, your whole chest and throat soften, and feel this relaxation spread deep within your chest. Finally feel how the tiny muscles of the bronchial tree become soft and relaxed. Keep this feeling of relaxation while you visualise yourself in perfect health, breathing easily and happily.

Repeat positive affirmations, whilst meditating or doing your daily activities. Remember to believe the affirmations, not just say them.

A useful visualisation is to see yourself happy and free to be yourself. Find out what it is that you love to do, what it is that defines you. Then visualise yourself doing it, whilst breathing easily, enjoying being here, and knowing that you have something very special to offer the world.

Release all negative emotions and limiting beliefs with the coaching programme.

Which therapies help?

Osteopathy and chiropractic help improve the function of the ribcage, diaphragm, secondary respiratory muscles, cervical and thoracic spine, which helps make breathing easier.

Cranial osteopathy also helps alleviate tension within the bronchial trees, lungs, thoracic fascia, spine and cranium. This is especially important if there has been a history of any birth trauma, and it is well known for its beneficial effect in the treatment of children.

Healing helps to balance the emotions.

Tibetan, ayurvedic and Chinese medicine and acupuncture help by treating the lungs and the immune system, as well as balancing the emotional energies.

Pilates is highly useful for restoring strength, balance and flexibility within the ribcage and spine, as well as helping to improve breathing ability.

Rolfing helps by breaking down fascial tension, which restricts the ribcage and thoracic spine.

Medical herbalism – Angelica helps prevent the build-up of phlegm and parsley, eucalyptus and Roman chamomile act as an antispasmodic.

Hypnotherapy, NLP and well-being coaching help by finding any underlying emotional triggers, unwanted negative emotions, or limiting decisions or beliefs and releasing them.

Useful Affirmations

"It is safe for me to be me and it is safe for me to be here."

"For every in-breath I breathe in love and happiness, and for every out-breath I share this love and happiness with others."

Warning: a severe asthma attack can be life-threatening and should always be treated in hospital. It is important to always be under the care of your medical doctor when you have asthma.

Babies Colic

This is defined as abdominal pain due to intestinal spasm. Colic often occurs in the evening, with the baby drawing the knees up to the chest, the abdomen distended and crying inconsolably. Colic is often thought to resolve at around 4 months of age, and there is natural improvement over time, but some babies continue to suffer until 6 months of age, and a few until 12 months.

What are the possible causes?

• Intolerance to formula, especially lactose, or something the mother is eating (such as dairy, wheat or nuts). A baby's digestive system does not mature until four to six months of age.
• Birth trauma, such as a quick or long labour, the use of forceps or ventouse, awkward birth position, or lying head down for a long period before birth are possible causes. These factors increase the strain placed on the baby's head and body as it descends through the birth canal, and often the baby experiences pain and discomfort after the birth. This can lead to compression of the nerve supplying the stomach as it exits from the area between the skull and the neck, as well as causing strain through the ribcage, thoracic spine, sacrum and the fascia in the gut.
• Swallowing air whilst eating can cause wind, which can lead to pain.
• Over feeding
• Spastic colon
• Reaction to vaccinations

What are the psychosomatic causes?

In a psychosomatic context colic may be an indication of being unsettled in the surroundings or feeling annoyed with something. Our digestive tract is highly dependent on our emotional state for its healthy functioning, so feelings of insecurity, irritation, impatience or frustration clearly can affect our digestion.

For a baby, the birth itself is a highly stressful experience, and it takes a while for any baby to get used to his surroundings. He has had a very closed and protected life in the womb and suddenly he is brought out into a world filled with stimulation, such as loud noises, bright lights, strange routines and lots of people. Some babies find this overwhelming and they become stressed which creates a negative impact on their immature digestive systems. Other babies may suffer from pain due to their birth, which is usually felt at the back of the head. The baby hates lying on her back and prefers being carried, rocked or being put in the car seat. Birth trauma can also be experienced around the stomach area due to tension within the ribcage and thoracic spine. This can make the baby highly stressed, frightened and angry, which affects her ability to digest food easily.

How can I help my baby in regards to the diet?

• Exclusively breast-feed your baby for the first six months.
• Make sure you are getting enough good, healthy food and drink, so that your body can easily produce nourishing breast milk. If you are depleted, then your milk will be depleted, too.
• If you breast-feed, avoid spicy food, coffee, chocolate, tea, brussel sprouts, garlic, onions, beans, dried fruit, bananas, large quantities of fresh fruit, carrots, broccoli or any other food that can cause wind, since these are passed on to the baby through the breast milk. Also avoid dairy, nut products and wheat.
• If formula feeding, consider changing to a goat milk formula. Goat milk is easier for the body to digest than cow milk. Soya milk formula may also be used, although watch for any sign of a soya intolerance. Special preparations of hydrolysed casein are available by prescription and can help babies with severe milk intolerance. To counteract any possible development of food sensitivities it may be wise to adopt a rotation formula diet, with five days of goat milk formula, five days of soya formula and five days of cow milk formula. If sensitivity is already present, such as an intolerance to cow milk, then this should be totally avoided.
• Feed your baby on demand. The crying may often be triggered by low blood sugar levels, since infants have not yet developed the ability to control this in the absence of food. Let your baby decide when she is hungry.

What else can I do to help?

Massage your baby's abdomen. Start at the bottom right hand corner of your baby's tummy (the baby's right), and with small, circular movements work your way up to the ribcage, massage across the stomach, just under the ribs and then down on the baby's left hand side. Keep doing this for about 5–20 minutes depending on how your baby is feeling. If your baby is suffering with constipation, then first massage the lower left hand corner of the abdomen (the baby's left) for a few minutes. There will be some faeces waiting to come out, and this needs to be loosened first, before you massage more faeces from the other areas of the intestines into this latter part of the colon.

A warm bath with a few drops of Roman chamomile or lavender oil may help to calm your baby, as well as help to reduce the spasm of the intestinal muscles.

Which supplements and herbs may be of help?

• Lactobacillus acidophilus supplements for the mother and child may help.
• Drink chamomile, fennel or ginger tea if you are breast-feeding. This helps to relax your baby's colon. If formula feeding, give 5–10 drops of fennel tincture to your baby daily.

How can I improve my baby's emotional, mental and spiritual health?

• Meditate whilst sitting next to your baby with your hand placed on your baby's tummy. Go inside your heart and connect with the deep love you feel for your child. Feel yourself opening up your heart and visualise how you extend this love to your baby though your hand.
• Keep a calm and relaxed atmosphere at home, with soft, gentle music playing.
• Make sure your baby gets enough sleep. Some babies are very inquisitive and will refuse to sleep as long as they can see what is going on, so you will need to reduce outside stimulation by using blackout curtains, or cover the buggy with a dark blanket.
• Babies are also soothed by movement that reminds them of the womb, when they were constantly being rocked to sleep, so taking your baby out for a walk will usually do the trick.

Which therapies help?

Cranial osteopathy is highly useful in the treatment of colic, especially when there are stresses and strains through the head, neck and body.

Baby massage helps to soothe the spasm of the intestines, and helps to alleviate tension in the gut.

Homeopathy – chamomilla 3x for babies

Healing – may be of great benefit for both the baby and the parents

Back Pain

This is a very common condition affecting about 80% of adults at some stage in their lives. Back pain can be acute or chronic. When acute, the onset is sudden, usually brought on by bending, lifting, twisting, falling or an accident. Unless the onset is traumatic, the cause of the pain usually lies in the daily habits of the affected person. The bending or lifting was only the final straw that broke the camel's back. Very often a history of vague and mild ache is reported, but these symptoms were dismissed or addressed by taking painkillers. Chronic pain develops slowly and lasts for a long period of time.

Why is it so painful?

When there is a strain or injury to a body structure, such as the joints, tendons or muscles, histamine and other chemicals are released by the damaged tissue which sets up an inflammatory reaction leading to swelling. This can increase the pressure on nearby structures causing pain, and the chemicals also stimulate the nerves that transmit pain. This is the body's way of trying to protect you from aggravating the injury, by making you stiffen up and feel pain as you place more strain on the injured area.

Unfortunately, it also restricts the circulation, which hinders important nutrients needed for healing from reaching the area. It is important to have appropriate treatment—such as osteopathy or chiropractic—to decrease the reaction, speed up the healing and allow the injured area to return to normal as soon as possible.

What are the causes of back pain?

There are many causes, starting with the fact that our bodies are designed for movement. We are meant to be doing daily exercise not leading a sedentary lifestyle.

Children have a more natural approach to fitness, they run around for a while, sit down, run around a little bit more and so on for all their waking hours (as any exhausted parent knows). Sadly, this stops the minute they start school and the pressures of life become apparent.

Other possible causes of back pain:
• Poor posture standing, sitting and walking
• Lack of exercise or the wrong type of exercise, such as breaststroke swimming (common cause of neck pain, headache, back and knee pain)
• Poor muscle tone, especially in back, abdomen, buttocks and legs
• Wearing high-heeled shoes
• Heavy physical work at home or in a job
• Spinal problems, with certain areas being either restricted or hyper-mobile causing increased stress on vulnerable joints
• Hips, knees, leg, ankle and feet misalignments
• Leg length discrepancy or scoliosis (when the spine is not straight)
• Disc injuries, facet joint problems, and muscle spasm
• Pregnancy or large bellies
• Digestive problems
• Dysfunctions of uterus or ovaries
• Arthritic conditions and osteoporosis
• Various types of bone disease and tumours
• Various types of organ disease, especially kidneys and pancreas
• Prostate problems
• Stress, both physical and emotional
• Difficult childbirth (especially if epidurals were used)
• Previous back surgery, which might have left scarring and fibrosis
• Previous use of myelograms (may cause an inflammation of the middle meningeal layer)
• Poor nutritional state

What are the psychosomatic causes?

In a psychosomatic context back pain can be an indicator of various emotional and mental issues. Upper back pain may indicate issues relating to the heart, such as lack of love, feeling unloved, or rejecting love. Pain in the middle back may be an indication of an inability to set boundaries and express ourselves. It can also relate to issues with guilt, or being stuck in the past. The lower back is our support system and our connection with the physical world. Pain there may indicate financial worries, lack of social support, relationship problems (such as bending over backwards to please), and sexual repression. We tend to store basic energy in the lower back, such as anger and resentment. The lower part of the spine is connected to the pelvis and the hips so it can also indicate an inability to let go and move forward in life.

How can I help myself?

See an osteopath or chiropractor immediately when you start to experience discomfort in your back. This will considerably shorten the time spent in pain.

If the back pain is acute, lie on your side with a cushion between your knees, so the spine is not twisted. Cold packs may be appropriate for the first few days. Keep the pack on for ten minutes, three to four times per day.

If acute, the pain will usually be worse in the morning because the inflammation has had time to build up, and sitting for prolonged periods of time will aggravate it due to increased pressure on affected areas. Best action is to lie down on your side to rest it, or move about gently. Let your pain guide you to what is appropriate.

When the pain has worn off and is more of a dull ache, staying active is often advisable.

Hot and cold hydrotherapy treatments (see **Therapies**) are useful when the pain is not acute. It helps to increase the circulation, which allows the body to heal quicker.

Change your lifestyle. Keep good posture when sitting, standing and walking. Always lift correctly. Start doing exercises for lower back and abdomen, to increase strength and flexibility. If you are overweight, change your eating and exercise habits, so that you take positive steps towards losing weight and maintaining it at a healthy level.

What should I avoid doing?

• Do not sleep on a very soft mattress and avoid sleeping on your stomach.
• Avoid wearing high-heeled shoes.
• Avoid painkillers unless absolutely necessary, because they will cut off the pain signals reaching the brain. It is more likely that you will injure yourself due to not feeling when your body is in a compromised position. If the pain is extremely bad, then taking painkillers before going to bed is okay, providing you keep still during the night.
• Do not drink coffee, tea or alcohol, since they decrease the amount of nutrients the body can absorb and prolong the healing time. Caffeine also increases the stress response in the body, which may contribute to increased muscular tonicity and pain.
• Quit smoking, since it decreases the circulation in the body and therefore makes it harder for all body tissues to maintain their health.

Which supplements and herbs help?

–Calcium and magnesium, since they have a relaxing action on the muscles
–Vitamin C with bioflavonoids to strengthen connective tissues
–A good vitamin B-complex for proper nerve function and bromelain as a digestive aid

–White willow bark is a natural pain reliever
–Herbal relaxants, such as passion flower, skull cap and Devil's claw helps as an anti-inflammatory
–Chamomile or thyme teas have muscle-relaxing actions

How can I improve my emotional, mental and spiritual health?

Look to see if any of the psychosomatic causes are true for you. If so, do something about it.

If stress is getting to you, make a daily habit to meditate, whilst visualising yourself in perfect health. A good exercise is to visualise your spine in perfect health. Focus on the area with the pain and feel the muscles soften, the ligaments relax, and the joints loosen. Then ask your unconscious mind what it needs you to pay attention to or learn, in order for your pain to go away.

Do the exercises in the coaching programme for releasing emotional pain held in the body or caused by unwanted states and behaviour, and for releasing negative emotions.

Once the pain has gone, what should I do?

Begin to look after yourself inside and out. Learn from the experience and accept that you need to look after your body in a way that you may not have done before. Make sure you have regular complementary treatments to keep yourself healthy and to prevent problems returning.

Exercise regularly, such as walking, yoga and Pilates. This helps to maintain your neuro-musculo-skeletal system in top condition.

When should I see my medical doctor?

If the pain in your back is also accompanied by

any of the following: nausea, vomiting, weight loss, fever, abdominal pain and pain down both arms or legs.

What requires immediate hospital attention?

- Numbness of buttocks and inner thighs
- Loss of bladder and bowel control
- Loss of erectile function

Which therapies help?

Osteopathy and chiropractic have been proven to be highly beneficial, especially in acute episodes of back pain.

Cranial osteopathy is particularly useful in long standing cases of back pain, or when there has been a history of trauma, such as an accident or fall.

Pilates is one of the most effective ways of helping to prevent back pain.

Massage is helpful especially in chronic cases of back pain.

Acupuncture helps by addressing the meridian and energy system. It is also an effective way of stopping the pain signals reaching the brain.

Kinesiology helps by addressing imbalances within the musculo-skeletal framework.

Healing helps when the pain is due to an emotional issue, or when the body is depleted.

NLP and hypnotherapy are useful when the pain is a symptom of a psychosomatic cause.

Useful affirmations

"It is now safe for me to move with ease through life."

"I am now able to fully support myself (and my family) doing something I love."

"I now let go of all the tension in my life."

Benign Prostatic Hypertrophy

The prostate gland is only present in males and secretes fluid that forms the main bulk of sperm. It is very common for it to enlarge after the age of forty, and it is then commonly known as benign prostatic hypertrophy (BPH).

What are the symptoms?

As the gland enlarges it starts to block the bladder outlet leading to symptoms such as an increased urgency to urinate, a feeling of not being able to empty the bladder fully, pain on urination, difficulty with stopping and starting, a need to urinate during the night and a decreased urine flow despite increased straining.

When should I contact a medical practitioner?

If you suffer from any of the symptoms listed above. You should see a doctor IMMEDIATELY if you also experience the following: recent weight loss, blood in the urine and/or fever and chills.

What are the causes?

- As men get older their testosterone levels fall, while other hormone levels rise such as prolactin, oestradiol and follicle stimulating hormones. This leads to an increased level of dihydrotestosterone within the prostate, which results in an overproduction of prostate cells leading to an enlarged prostate.
- Prolactin production can be enhanced by stress and beer drinking thereby aggravating this process. A deficiency in zinc and vitamin B6 will do the same.
- Other factors that may predispose to this condition are a diet rich in refined, fried and fatty foods, coffee, tea, and alcohol.

• Lack of essential fatty acids in the diet.
• Lack of exercise.
• Pelvic congestion, such as constipation, poor blood circulation, increased toxicity of the blood due to poor eating habits and poor elimination processes.
• Lack of abdominal tone.
• Infection, such as gonorrhoea.
• Pesticides and heavy metals.
• Very high stress levels.

What are the psychosomatic causes?

In a psychosomatic context problems with the prostate may indicate deeply held fears relating to our masculinity and our ability to perform sexually. When it becomes enlarged and starts to affect the bladder obstructing the flow of urine, it may indicate that we are being unable to express our frustration and negative emotions relating to these fears.

How is BPH treated?

Very often BPH is conventionally treated with surgery, but this can lead to several complications. Natural treatments have shown to be very effective in the treatment of BPH and can also offer protection from ever developing it.

How can I help in regards to the diet?

• A detox may be indicated, such as only apples or grapes for 3-7 days. This is a very effective way of getting rid of a build-up of toxins, but should only be undertaken under the supervision of a naturopathic physician.
• Increase consumption of vegetables, fruits, brown rice, pasta and bread.
• Increase intake of fatty fish, olive oil, nuts, almonds, sunflower, pumpkin and sesame seeds for their essential fatty acid content.
• Increase intake of pumpkin seeds, nuts, garlic, onions, brown rice, carrots and Brewer's yeast for their zinc content. A golden rule is to eat half a cup of pumpkin seeds and three almonds daily for their essential fatty acid and zinc content.
• Eat soya based foods regularly, since these are rich in phytosterols, which seems to both protect against prostate cancer and reduce the symptoms of benign prostate hypertrophy.
• Eat organic as much as possible and drink plenty of filtered water.

What should I avoid?

Avoid refined carbohydrates, fried and fatty foods, coffee, tea, alcohol and cigarettes.

How else can I improve my physical health?

• If an infection is present, such as gonorrhoea, it must be treated with antibiotics. Supplement with lactobacillus acidophilus to restore the gut flora, but be sure to take the lactobacillus at least 3 hours after the antibiotics.
• Hot and cold sitz baths are used to increase the circulation and stimulate the pelvic organs. (This should never be done in the acute stages).
• A hot compress or sitz bath can be used to decrease the pressure on the urethra and allow full emptying of the bladder. This should never be used if an acute inflammation or infection is present.
• Avoid having interrupted intercourse, prolonged intercourse or long periods of abstinence.

Which supplements and herbs help?

• Supplement with essential fatty acids, such as flax seed oil capsules and cod liver oil daily. Also take a tablespoon of olive oil once per day.
• Supplement with a good B-complex, extra B6, antioxidant (vitamin A, C and E), zinc, seleni-

um and garlic capsules daily.

• Psyllium husks or whole linseeds should be used to aid in proper bowel movements, since constipation will increase the discomfort felt due to the enlarged prostate.

• Various herbs may be of help, such as saw palmetto, stinging nettle, and cernilton (extract of flower pollen). See a medical herbalist for a more detailed assessment.

How can I improve my emotional, mental and spiritual health?

Meditate or practice some other form of relaxation daily. This is vital since stress increases the prolactin production, which leads to an increase in dihydrotestosterone.

If you feel any negative emotions relating to your sexuality and/or masculinity, then deal with them. With the aid of the coaching programme find out your values for relationships and sexuality, any negative emotions and limiting beliefs you may have relating to these areas, and release these with the exercises outlined in this book. After you have done this, then write down your new values for the same areas. These values should now be aligned and positive, supporting you in experiencing happiness, harmony and balance within these two areas of your life.

If there is anyone you have any unresolved issues with, then do the forgiveness exercise. This will allow you to let go of the past, which will free up energy that instead can be used to heal your body.

When you meditate, ask your prostate what it wants you to pay attention to, know or learn in order for it to get better. Ask what is the highest wisdom for you. Then act on this guidance.

A good meditation to do is the following: Go within to the inner stillness. Place your awareness in your heart and feel the loving energy

there. Then send this love to your prostate, keep sending it as much love as you possibly can. Do this exercise every day.

Visualise seeing yourself in front of you. See yourself as the man you desire to be, filled with all the good qualities you desire to have. What does he look like? Float inside this ideal picture of yourself and feel the feelings he has, and look through the world with his eyes. What feelings does he have? How does he perceive the world? Then float back inside the present you again. Now ask this ideal version of yourself what you need to know or learn in order for you to become him. Make sure you get this information and then feel yourself merge with this ideal you, so that you take on his wisdom and energy.

Which therapies help?

Medical herbalism has several herbs that can be of benefit. Always see a practitioner for specific advice.

Tibetan, ayurvedic and Chinese medicine and acupuncture are effective treatments in helping the body come back into balance again, as much as is possible.

Osteopathic and chiropractic treatment help by assisting to reduce pelvic congestion, treating any underlying constipation and restoring proper nerve, blood and lymphatic supply to the prostate and other related structures.

Acupressure, shiatzu and reflexology assist the body by stimulating pressure points relating to the prostate, digestive tract and adrenal glands.

Healing is beneficial by balancing the emotions and energy levels within your body and mind.

Homeopathic remedies such as sabal serrulata (when there is a feeling of coldness in the sexual organs, difficulty passing urine, and frequent need to urinate during the night); chimaphila umbellata (when there is urine retention due to enlarged prostate); and clematis (when the urine is passed in drops with dribbling afterwards). Many other remedies are suitable, but please see a practitioner for appropriate advice.

Aromatherapy helps by using specific oils to balance the emotions, as well as assisting through massage for releasing tension held within the pelvic region.

NLP, hypnotherapy and well-being coaching help to assist you in releasing negative emotions and limiting beliefs, reducing stress levels and changing unwanted and unhelpful states and behaviours.

Useful affirmations

"I am loveable just as I am."

"It is safe for me to grow old with grace."

"Every age contains within it its own love, wisdom and beauty."

"Only love matters. It does not matter which form or shape it takes, only that it is made with pure love."

Bronchitis and Pneumonia

Bronchitis is an inflammation of the bronchial tree, usually preceded by an upper respiratory tract infection. It may be acute or chronic. When acute, there is sudden onset of fever, chills, chest pain, coughing, breathing difficulty and fatigue. When chronic, it is more of a constant irritation of the bronchial tree, with a persistent cough with sputum, breathing difficulty and wheezing, but without any fever and chills. Pneumonia is an inflammation of the lungs, which is also due to an infection or irritation. It can be a highly deadly disease, especially in the elderly. It has very similar symptoms and signs as acute bronchitis, except that the sputum will possibly be stained with blood.

What are the causes?

Bronchitis and pneumonia are usually due to an infection, such as a cold or the flu, which often is viral, and sometimes bacterial. Antibiotics are definitely recommended in severe bacterial pneumonia, but have no effect in viral pneumonia, and usually are not needed in bronchitis. Unfortunately antibiotics are often used, leading to disruption of a healthy gut flora, increased development of antibiotic resistant bacteria leading to 'super-bugs', and over growth of candida albicans.

What causes an infection to take hold?

• Poor diet, which is high in sugar, refined foods, coffee, tea or alcohol, and low in fruits and vegetables.
• Suppression of previous colds and flu. For example, when you have a cold with a fever, and you don't want to stay home from work, you take a cold or flu remedy to help you through

the day. You feel better whilst the remedy is working, and assume you can go to work. Where do you think the energy will come from? Your body does not want to be active. It wants to stay at home and rest, and when you don't, you exhaust your energy reserves and set up an opportunity for other infections to take hold.

• Food allergies leading to immuno-suppression
• Poor elimination, including improper functioning of the digestive tract leading to constipation, sluggish liver, poor skin function and circulation
• Smoking and smoky environments
• Asthma, emphysema or bronchial constriction
• Chemical and heavy metal pollutants
• Lack of exercise
• Exercise in very cold climates where the bronchial tree and lungs are filled with icy cold air. This is particularly common in athletes in northern countries such as Sweden and Finland.
• Spinal dysfunction in the thoracic spine leading to decreased function of the bronchial tree and lungs
• Poor immune system, due to illness, previous infections, immuno-suppressive drugs or severe stress
• HIV, chronic infections, kidney failure, drug and alcohol abuse

What are the psychosomatic causes?

In the psychosomatic context bronchitis may indicate repressed emotions, such as anger, frustration and sadness. This may be due to our inability to express ourselves, causing inner tension, or due to a difficult family environment. Since we need to breathe in the air from our environment, there may be something we do not like, and therefore the bronchial tree becomes irritated. The lungs are our first point of separation from the inner world in the womb, because as we breathe the first breath we start our life as separate from our mother. Therefore problems with the lungs may relate to our inability to be independent, or a feeling of being tired of 'doing it on our own', a feeling of being tired of life. Since it is in the area of the heart it may also be due to unhealed emotions felt in the heart.

How can I help improve in regards to the diet?

Increase the function of the immune system (see **Immune System**).

A juice fast may be beneficial in case of bronchitis. Only use diluted juices and do not do this unless you are under the supervision of a qualified naturopath.

For bronchitis, increase consumption of onions, garlic, and chili and cayenne peppers since they aid in opening up the bronchial passages.

What should I avoid?

Avoid all dairy products (mucous forming), sugar, refined foods, coffee, tea and alcohol.

How else can I improve my physical health?

• Bed rest
• Hot and cold packs (see **Therapies**) to the trunk and throat to stimulate the circulation and improve the function of the trachea, lungs and thymus gland
• Hot and cold showers to stimulate the circulation. Alternatively have a sauna followed by a cold shower, then repeat
• Inhalation of olbas oil, pine needles and eucalyptus is very good to improve lung and bronchial function
• Breathing exercises, especially diaphragmatic breathing
• Postural drainage of the mucous. First do a hot chest pack, and then lie over a table on your

stomach so that your head and chest are hanging over the edge. Let someone do percussion (gentle tapping) over your ribcage to stimulate drainage of the mucous secretions. Have a bucket underneath so that you can spit out all the mucous. This will help to clear the lungs. When you do this with children, have them sitting upright in your lap, whilst percussing gently on their ribcage.

• Castor oil packs (see **Therapies**) to the liver once a week to aid in the elimination process and improve immune function.

Which supplements and herbs help?

• During the first days of infection it is highly beneficial to take regular low doses of vitamin C (250 mg every 4 hours).

• Beta-carotene (converts into vitamin A) is important for the healthy functioning of lung tissue and mucous membranes. Vitamin E, C and zinc also aid in tissue healing.

• B-complex may be needed.

• Echinacea, propolis and goldenseal are potent stimulators of the immune system.

• Other various herbs can help, such as liquorice, wild-cherry bark, horehound, sundew and lobelia. See a medical herbalist for further advice.

• Bromelain has shown to be effective in the treatment of upper respiratory infections. In chronic bronchitis it has shown to suppress the cough and to reduce the viscosity of the sputum (1).

How can I improve my emotional, mental and spiritual health?

It is much better to let your feelings be heard, than to bottle them up. Learn to express yourself in a calm and respectful manner, so that you are being honest with others about your feelings without fuelling any anger. All you can do is to be true to yourself and responsible for your own

emotional well-being. It is up to others how they respond to your honesty as long as what you say is coming from your heart and with a sense of detachment from wanting a specific outcome.

Have you got clear boundaries with people in your life, or do you let others walk all over you? What positive steps can you take so that you achieve a sense of peace, calm and happiness in your environment, both at home and at work?

With the coaching programme release all your negative emotions, pain held in the body and caused by unwanted states and behaviours.

What is it your bronchitis/pneumonia wants you to pay attention to, so that if you were to pay attention to it, it would heal?

Practice gentle breathing exercises (breathe in to a count of four and out to a count of four in a relaxed manner). This will help your lungs to improve their health, but it will also help you to release stress, tension and negative emotions, whilst stilling your mind and enabling you to connect with your spiritual self and inner wisdom.

Visualise yourself in perfect health. Feel how you breathe in health, vitality and joy, and as you breathe out you let these positive qualities flow to all the cells in your whole being—body, mind and spirit.

Which therapies help?

Osteopathy and cranial osteopathy help by improving the function of the immune system, as well as releasing restrictions and tension held in the neck, thoracic spine, ribcage, lungs, bronchial tree and diaphragm.

Tibetan, ayurvedic and Chinese medicine and acupuncture help to relax tension and stimulate healing through the use of herbs, massage and acupuncture.

Reflexology, acupressure and shiatzu help by stimulating pressure points relating to the lungs and bronchial trees.

Medical herbalism has many useful herbs.

Homeopathic remedies are often useful.

Healing helps to balance the emotions, release blocked tension and restore energy.

NLP, hypnotherapy and well-being coaching help by releasing past negative emotions and mental blockages, which are draining the immune system.

If you suspect pneumonia you must go to your medical doctor immediately.

useful affirmations

"It is safe for me to express myself fully and honestly."

"As I release the old I am able to breathe in and fully experience the new."

"I am an eternal being filled with love and light. I now relax and trust life."

candida

This is an overgrowth of candida albicans, which is a yeast-like fungus in the body. When the body's good bacteria (lactobacillus and bifidus) have decreased, due to lowered immune system or after taking antibiotics, this yeast can take over, sending out toxins that interfere with a range of various systems of the body, mainly the gastrointestinal, nervous, endocrine and immune systems.

What are the common symptoms?

Chronic fatigue, thrush, bloating, stomach cramps, gas, altered bowel function, rectal itching, frequent urinary tract infections, prostatitis, PMS, depression, anxiety, poor concentration, lowered immune function, loss of libido, respiratory problems, recurrent skin and/or nail fungus infections (such as athlete's foot), allergies and chemical sensitivities. The affected individual often has cravings for the foods that aggravate the condition, such as sugar, bread and alcohol.

How can chronic candidiasis lead to 'leaky gut syndrome'?

This is due to the candida damaging the gut lining, which creates large holes in the wall. This can allow protein molecules from undigested food to leak through, which can lead to allergies.

Who are most likely to suffer?

Women are up to eight times more likely to suffer than men, which may be due to the birth-control pill, the effect of oestrogen and an increased incidence of antibiotic use. Antibiotic use may have contributed to an increase of common conditions affecting children, such as allergies, hyperactivity and frequent infections (usually ears and chest).

Possible causes

- Prolonged, or frequent, antibiotic use
- Altered bowel flora and decreased digestive secretions
- Poor dietary habits, especially high sugar intake, in which candida thrives
- Alcohol intake, since this feeds the yeast
- Poor absorption of B-vitamins, especially B6 and biotin
- Oral contraceptive use and cortico-steroid use
- Anti-ulcer medications, such as Tagamet (cimetidine) and Zantac (ranitidine)
- Low immune function
- Diabetes, gallbladder problems, cancer and hypothyroidism
- Impaired liver function
- Food and environmental allergies

What are the psychosomatic causes?

In the psychosomatic context, a yeast infection of the vagina or gastro-intestinal tract may be relating to unexpressed emotions, such as anger, sadness, fear and guilt and our inability to digest and deal with these emotions. When the vagina is affected it may indicate unresolved problems dealing with our sexuality, such as past abuse, inability to enjoy sex, or not trusting a sexual partner. It may indicate an issue of not wanting to give of oneself.

How can I help in regards to the diet?

Increase intake of all non-sweet vegetables, legumes, fish, poultry and whole grain.

Since candida often is linked to thrush, it is useful to drink 3–4 glasses of pure cranberry juice (not the drink, since it contains sugar) per day. If pure juice cannot be found, cranberry tablets can be taken instead. Blueberries are also beneficial. Both of these berries help to keep the urinary tract healthy by preventing bacteria adhering to the walls of the bladder and urethra.

What should I avoid?

- Totally avoid the use of antibiotics, steroids and birth control pills unless there is an absolute necessity on medical grounds.
- Avoid any type of sugar (fruit sugar, honey, brown sugar, white sugar, alcohol), yeast or mould (wine, beer, smoked and pickled food, fermented foods, certain breads, cheeses, dried fruits, melons, concentrated orange juice, raisins, overripe foods and peanuts) and dairy products (due to milk-sugar 'lactose').
- Avoid coffee and tea.
- Avoid all foods that are a known allergen, since these weaken the immune system, which makes it easier for the candida to grow.
- Decrease the intake of corn, parsnip and potatoes due to their sugar content.

Which fruits can I eat in small amounts?

Apples, berries, cherries and pears

Which supplements and herbs help?

- Liver support is important throughout the treatment, since the liver has to filter the toxins that the candida releases as it dies off. If proper support is not given, there will be a worsening of symptoms and it may be difficult to continue with the treatment. For optimal health of this important organ it is best to avoid any alcohol, drastically cut the intake of sugar, fat, pollutants and pesticides. Milk thistle, especially silymarin, is a very potent liver detoxifier. Lipotropic factors, such as lecithin, choline, betaine and methionine help to promote the flow of fat and bile to and from the liver. See a naturopath or medical herbalist for more advice.

• Lactobacillus acidophilus and bifidus will help to control the yeast via manufacture of biotin (a B-vitamin). It also helps to restore the healthy gut flora. A B-complex may be needed. Make sure it is not yeast based. A high potency multivitamin and mineral is also recommended.

• Take psyllium husks to bind the toxins from the candida in the gut.

• Increase the function of the immune system by taking anti-oxidant supplements (vitamin A, C, E, zinc and selenium). Also complement this with echinacea and goldenseal.

• Take daily high doses of garlic, since it has an effective anti-fungal effect.

• Use cinnamon, rosemary, thyme and ginger as much as possible, since they contain candida-killing substances. Enteric-coated peppermint capsules and oregano have been shown to reduce candida albicans overgrowth (2). However, peppermint capsules must be given only when a correct diagnosis has been made, since it can damage the gut in an individual suffering from an inflammatory bowel disease.

• German chamomile is good at killing candida.

• Pau d'arco and clove tea are useful due to their anti-bacterial and anti fungal properties.

How can I improve my emotional, mental and spiritual health?

Look at your values for relationships and family (see Chapter One on values in the coaching programme). Do you have any limiting beliefs, which are restricting you from experiencing happiness in these areas? Do you have any issues regarding sex and your femininity?

With the help of the coaching programme release all negative emotions, limiting beliefs, emotional pain held in the body and caused by unwanted states and behaviours. Do the forgiveness exercise in relation to all your previous partners, your present partner and your parents.

Meditate daily, so that you start to experience the deep inner stillness, happiness and light within you. When you feel this inner happiness let it flow to every cell of your body, until your whole being is radiating health, happiness and light. This sends very clear signals to your unconscious mind that this is now what is required of it. Your immune system will benefit greatly, and it will be much easier for your body to experience a profound state of health.

Ask the candida what it wants you to pay attention to, know or learn for it to heal?

Each one of us has something beautiful within that we are meant to share with the world. In which ways do you allow your inner beauty and love to shine forth? What steps can you take to increase that?

Which therapies help?

Medical herbalism – there are several herbs that can help to address candidiasis, such as goldenseal, oregano oil, thyme oil and peppermint oil. See a qualified practitioner to determine exactly which herbs are most suitable for your treatment.

Homeopathy – there is a remedy for candida albicans. Always see a practitioner for appropriate advice.

Aromatherapy – a good therapist will be able to find oils that help to de-stress the mind, which will have a beneficial effect on the whole immune system.

Tibetan, ayurvedic and Chinese medicine and acupuncture are excellent for addressing any imbalances within the gastro-intestinal tract and for improving the immune system, both of which are needed for successful treatment of candida overgrowth.

Osteopathy and chiropractic help to improve the functioning of the gastro-intestinal tract and liver by working on the nerve and blood supply to these organs. Tension held in the fascia surrounding the gut can also be released. In this way the general health of the gastro-intestinal tissue is improved and it is easier for the individual to fight off the candida overgrowth.

Reflexology, shiatzu and acupressure help by stimulating pressure points related to the digestive tract, liver and adrenal glands.

Kinesiology helps by establishing if there are any underlying food allergies.

Healing helps to balance the emotions and the energy within the body.

Yoga and Pilates help to improve the functioning of the spine, so the nerve and blood supply to the whole gut can function optimally. Useful exercises are the Spinal Twist, Pelvic Bridge, the Cat and the Mermaid.

Hypnotherapy, NLP and well-being coaching – if you suspect any underlying emotional issues then these therapies are excellent in finding the true cause, releasing it and helping you move forward in a healthy and balanced way.

Useful affirmations:

"It is safe for me to love and trust myself and others."

"It is safe for me to share my innermost feelings with others."

"I am filled with light and love, and as I share this light and love with others, it returns to me multiplied."

Chronic Fatigue Syndrome

Chronic fatigue syndrome is a complex illness that is becoming more common. It has a wide range of symptoms, such as sore throat, chronic fatigue, swollen lymph glands, aching muscles, joint pain, headaches, low-grade fever, depression, problems with concentration, confusion, stomach pain and recurrent episodes of infection. The whole immune system seems to be compromised, giving rise to these varied symptoms.

What causes it?

The cause is unknown, but many theories have suggested that it is due to a chronic Epstein-Barr virus (EBV) infection. Most of us carry antibodies in our blood to the EBV from a previous infection, usually in childhood. It belongs to the herpes family, which include herpes simplex (type 1 and 2), varicella zoster (chicken pox and in its reactivated form, shingles), cytomegalovirus and pseudorabies virus. These viruses produce lifelong infections that lie dormant until they have a chance to resurface. This happens when the immune system is not working properly, which can be due to a variety of reasons. An elevation of the EBV is also seen in a number of conditions, such as AIDS, multiple sclerosis, ankylosing spondylitis, rheumatoid arthritis, systemic lupus erythematosus, kidney dysfunction, lymphatic tumours and chemotherapy.

What other causes have been suggested?

Other causes may be combined infections, such as from yeast, parasites, bacterial and viral; vaccination toxicity; genetic susceptibility; food allergies/sensitivities; previous accidents, such as whiplash injuries; and anything else that depletes the immune system.

What are the psychosomatic causes?

Chronic fatigue syndrome (CFS) may indicate a loss of purpose or direction in life, a deep feeling of wanting to withdraw from life's responsibilities and demands. It may also indicate an individual who has been forcing herself to keep up the same pace even when her body starts to give warning signals that all is not well. Eventually there is no more fuel left in the body and the affected person totally collapses, drained physically, emotionally, mentally and spiritually. It invariably leads to exhaustion of the adrenal glands.

How can I help in regards to my diet?

Eat plenty of fruits, vegetables, soya, tofu and fish. Drink 6–8 glasses of water per day.

It is often necessary to go on an elimination diet to exclude any food sensitivities, and it may be needed to properly detoxify the body, since this would effectively reduce many obstacles that prevent healing. Only do this under the supervision of a qualified practitioner, such as a naturopath.

What should I avoid?

Avoid refined food, red meat, excess dairy products, sugar, colourings, additives, coffee, tea and alcohol. Large caffeine consumption leads to adrenal exhaustion, which in turn can lead to chronic fatigue.

Which supplements and herbs help?

• Lactobacillus acidophilus and bifidus help the gut to function better, thereby improving health.

• Essential fatty acids are necessary, such as flax seed oil (omega 3 and 6), evening primrose oil (omega 6), and fish oil (omega 3).

• If sleep is disturbed, supplementation of calcium and magnesium 30–45 minutes before bedtime will aid relaxation. A hot soya drink enriched with calcium can be used as well (soya is naturally high in magnesium). Magnesium supplementation is important, since a magnesium deficiency can have similar symptoms as chronic fatigue syndrome.

• Milk thistle, liquorice root and artichoke are very good for helping the function of the liver.

• Echinacea may be needed to improve the immune system, and ginseng can help the body to better cope with stress. If depression is present St John's wort may be suitable. Consult a medical herbalist before taking any herbs, since the requirements and suitability vary from person to person.

How else can I improve my physical health?

• Improve the immune system (see **Immune System**).

• Do lymphatic exercises. Stand upright. Go up on your tiptoes at the same time as you swing your arms behind you, breathing out as much as you can. Come down to stand flat on your soles, whilst taking a deep breath in and bringing your arms first down and then up straight in front of you. Then again go up on your tiptoes, swinging the arms fully back behind you, whilst you breathe out fully. Do this 20–30 times, at least 4–5 times per day. This will encourage a healthy functioning of the lymphatic system.

• Brush your skin with a dry loofah in circular movements up towards your heart before having a shower.

• Have hot and cold showers to stimulate circulation and aid elimination.

• Do weekly castor oil packs (see **Therapies**) to the liver to aid elimination.

• Do hot and cold packs to your spine to improve circulation to all organs.

Which exercises may be of help?

Yoga and Pilates – when you suffer with CFS the last thing you think about is exercise. However, it is vital that the body is still being used in a gentle and effective way. Several yoga and Pilates exercises help to stimulate the immune system, such as the Spinal Twist, the Cat and breathing exercises.

Walking daily

Swimming (back stroke and crawl only)

How can I improve my emotional, mental and spiritual health?

Learn to say 'no'. Let go of the need to want to do it all, and create better boundaries around you, so that you only do those tasks you feel happy doing.

What is within you that you long to bring forth and share with the world? What would you be and do if you could be and do anything you want? What would your day, week and life be like? Answer these questions, and you will start to reveal your authentic self, which longs to share itself with life.

How much do you allow yourself to fill your days doing things that give you joy and pleasure? What steps can you take to increase this in your life?

Find out your values for health and living, and do the appropriate exercises for it in the coaching programme.

With the aid of the coaching programme release all negative emotions, limiting beliefs and do the forgiveness exercise for all key people in your life, as well your CFS.

Practice meditation and breathing exercises

daily. These have been used for thousands of years as a way to control, restore and improve the energy levels in the body. One useful exercise is to sit comfortably with your back straight, and focus your gaze on a spot straight in front of you. Keep focusing on this spot as you also expand your awareness to the periphery (called peripheral vision), whilst breathing in through your nose and out through your mouth in a ratio of 1:1 (breathing in to a count of four and breathing out to a count of four). Do this for 5–10 minutes, and you will be amazed how quickly it has a positive effect on you.

A useful therapy is to visualise red energy from the earth rising up through your feet, up your legs, through your abdomen and spine, into your neck and up to your head. Then visualise your head opening up and let universal white or golden energy flow from the top of your head, through your neck, spine, abdomen, legs and feet. Keep visualising and feeling these two sets of energy currents flowing through you, until you feel thoroughly energised. Then picture yourself in perfect and radiant health.

Visualise your chronic fatigue in front of you. Send it as much love as you possibly can. See the love penetrate through every layer of its being, and see how it starts to radiate a beautiful golden, healing light. Keep doing this until the healing feels complete. Then rest in this peacefulness for a few moments before opening your eyes.

Which therapies help?

Osteopathy and chiropractic help because misalignment in the physical framework can affect the immune system negatively. By addressing this misalignment, proper nerve, blood and lymphatic functions may be restored which help the body to heal. Cranial osteopathic techniques help to balance the central nervous system.

Tibetan, ayurvedic and Chinese medicine help greatly to balance the body's energy systems and promote the functioning of the immune system. They do so through the use of acupuncture, massage and herbs.

Medical herbalism has several excellent herbs for restoring healthy energy levels in the body. You need to see a qualified practitioner, so that you get herbs that are specifically suited for your requirements.

Homeopathic remedies are useful. See a practitioner for specific advice.

Reflexology, shiatzu and acupressure help by stimulating pressure points relating to the immune system and adrenal glands.

Healing helps by balancing the emotions and the energy levels within the body.

Hypnotherapy, NLP and well-being coaching help by addressing and releasing unresolved emotional issues and negative thought patterns, such as limiting beliefs and decisions. An enormous amount of energy becomes available to the body, which was previously used to repress these. It also improves balance within your life, creating better coping strategies and setting up positive goals for the future.

Useful affirmations

"I have all the energy I need within me."

"For every task that comes my way, the energy is also supplied."

"Life is wonderful and it is to be lived fully."

"I am now creating the life of my dreams."

"It is now safe for me to live as my authentic self."

Colds, Flu and Sinusitis

Colds and flu are caused by a viral infection of the upper respiratory tract. The flu is far more severe than a cold, and a new strain of the flu virus appears each year, and usually occurs in epidemics just as the first real signs of winter set in. Sinusitis is an inflammatory process in the sinuses due to bacterial, viral, fungal or allergic reactions.

Colds and Flu

The symptoms can be aching muscles, swollen lymph glands, headache, nasal congestion, sore throat, sneezing, coughing, tiredness, diarrhoea and fever. A cold will develop gradually, while the flu has a rapid onset.

Can having a cold be a good thing?

Yes, because a common cold is the body's way of cleansing and getting rid of waste products that have accumulated with time. It is normal, healthy and desirable to have one or two episodes of a short lasting cold per year.

When can having a cold be a sign of a low immune system?

When you have more than two colds per year, or if it is prolonged over a period of weeks or months. Never having a cold indicates that the body's elimination process is not working properly, and this can lead to serious ill health later on in life.

Sinusitis

An acute bacterial sinus infection is often preceded by an upper respiratory tract infection, such as a common cold. In chronic sinusitis it is usually due to an allergic reaction or an underlying dental infection.

What can predispose to sinusitis?

- Food allergens (especially milk)
- Poor diet
- Low immune function
- Dental problems and previous dental work causing strain within the cranial vault
- Cervical (neck) and upper thoracic restrictions, leading to poor nerve, blood and lymphatic function
- Various obstructions, such as deviated septum and polyps
- Poor bowel function and liver congestion
- Stress leading to adrenal exhaustion and decreased immune system
- Previous falls and injuries to the head may have set up a dysfunction in the areas where the sinuses reside: frontal (forehead), ethmoid (between eyes and the nose), sphenoid (behind eyes) and maxillary (cheek bones).

What are the psychosomatic causes?

A cold may be a sign that we need time out to nurture ourselves and look at what may be bothering us. It may be an indication of blocked tears, or emotional issues that need to be released. It is the body's way of cleansing us and trying to bring our body and mind back into balance. Flu is a very powerful way of cleansing the body from a build up of toxins, and due to its shear intensity it is forcing us to stop and rest. It may indicate that our body and mind need a rest or that we feel helpless about something outside our control. Sinusitis may indicate problems expressing blocked emotions or thoughts, or blocked tears.

How can I help in regards to my diet?

- Drink diluted fruit juices. If not diluted the sugar content will decrease the white blood cell count, which will decrease the immune function. If you are hungry eat only fresh fruits and steamed vegetables.
- Eat plenty of vegetables (especially onions and garlic), fruits, pumpkin, sesame and sunflower seeds.
- Eat plenty of seaweed and fish for its zinc content.
- Drink lots of filtered water.
- The most important help is prevention. So improve your immune system (see **Immune System**) by eating a healthy diet, practising regular forms of relaxation, exercising moderately, avoid smoking and keep alcohol and caffeine to a minimum.

What should I avoid?

- Avoid eating when you have the flu. Animals and children refuse food during an elimination process, since the body does not need any more material to deal with.
- Avoid dairy products (milk, yoghurt, cheese), since they are mucous forming.
- Avoid sugar, since glucose and vitamin C fight with each other for the transport sites into the white blood cells. This results in lowered vitamin C levels and therefore a reduced function of the white blood cells.
- Avoid common food allergens.

What else can I do to help?

- Do not suppress any symptoms. They are there for a reason—to make you rest. Do not suppress a fever unless it is above 40 degrees C (104 degrees F). Never give aspirin to a child or teenager who has a viral cold or flu, since this combination has been linked to Reye's syndrome, a very serious liver disease seen in young people.

• Rest and sleep are probably the most important tools for helping the immune system recover.

• Hot and cold packs to the throat are very good for sore throats and to stimulate the function of the thymus gland.

• Epsom salt baths encourage elimination

• Hot mustard footbaths increase elimination

• Make sure your feet are always warm.

• For congested heads and sinuses put eucalyptus, clove, pine and thyme oil in a pot of boiling water to make a steam. Then place your face just over the pot and cover with a towel. Stay in there for 4–5 minutes constantly taking deep breaths to really fill the lungs. This can also be done for children. Then place them on your lap, and cover both of you with a big sheet.

• For sore throats try gargling with warm water, honey and lemon juice.

Which supplements and herbs help?

• Take at least 3–5 garlic capsules a day. If you can tolerate it, eat 2–3 crushed raw cloves of garlic.

• Vitamin C, A, E and beta-carotene are all beneficial.

• Zinc lozenges or tablets help the immune system greatly.

• Lactobacillus acidophilus and bifidus are very good for aiding the function of the intestines by restoring friendly gut bacteria.

• Echinacea should be used throughout the illness.

• Goldenseal is a good anti-viral herb, astralgus is a potent immune stimulator and wild indigo helps to improve the immune system.

• Propolis (bee pollen) has also shown to aid in the recovery of a cold or flu. Do not take if you are allergic to propolis (sometimes seen in hay fever).

• Bromelain has helped patients with acute sinusitis (54).

How can I improve my emotional, mental and spiritual health?

• Meditate on your condition. What does it need you to pay attention to, so that if you were to pay attention to it your condition would go away?

• Find out the emotional content of your condition by doing the meditation for releasing emotional pain held in the body.

• Do the forgiveness exercise in relation to everyone you feel any negativity towards.

• Meditate and practice breathing exercises daily. This will aid you in gently balancing your emotions and thoughts on a regular basis.

• Visualise yourself in perfect health. See how your heart pumps out fresh, nutritious blood to every cell in your body, so that they get the energy they need. Then see how the blood removes waste products, which are no longer needed. Open up the soles of your feet and drain these waste products away from your body and mind, through the soles of your feet, and into the earth, where they become purified. Keep doing this until you feel thoroughly cleansed. Then open up the top of your head and draw in universal light. Feel your body and mind become re-energised by this light. Finally allow yourself to rest.

Which therapies help?

During an acute phase of flu it is best to rest and support the body through the use of herbs, vitamins and minerals. Once the acute phase of a flu virus has passed and there is no temperature present, physical treatment is appropriate. You can usually have treatment during a cold or sinusitis.

Medical herbalism has many useful herbs.

Tibetan, ayurvedic and Chinese medicine are beneficial for restoring well-being and energy in a depleted body and mind.

Osteopathy and chiropractic help after an infection as a way to restore neuro-musculo-skeletal balance, which has a beneficial effect on the immune system. Cranial osteopathy is especially useful for sinusitis as it can gently manipulate the cranial bones to aid drainage of the sinuses.

Reflexology, acupressure and shiatzu help by stimulating the function of the immune system.

Homeopathy has several remedies, which may be of benefit, such as belladonna, dulcamara and pulsatilla.

NLP, hypnotherapy and well-being coaching help release negative emotions and limiting beliefs, which are depleting you.

useful affirmations

"Life is perfect just as it is."

"It is now safe for me to let go of the old and embrace the new."

"I now allow my emotions to be expressed and released safely and gently."

"My mind is filled with peace and harmony."

Common Female Conditions

The following conditions are related to the hormone production, reproductive system and general well-being of a woman. They are covered together, since the treatments are very similar.

Cervical Dysplasia

This is the development of abnormal cells of the uterine cervix, and is the second most common form of cancer of the female reproductive tract.

How is it diagnosed?

It is diagnosed by a Pap smear test and gynaecological examination. There are four classes of a Pap smear test: class 1 has normal cells, class 2–4 have pre-cancerous cells, the severity increasing with the number, class 5 has cancerous cells. Cervical dysplasia is usually thought of as a pre-cancerous lesion, and it is estimated that about 30 to 50% of women with cervical dysplasia later develop cervical cancer, which can be in situ (in the cervix) or invasive (spreading to other structures). In situ usually occurs in women around the age of thirty and invasive

cervical carcinoma in women in their mid-forties and fifties. Invasive carcinoma is decreasing, probably due to the Pap smear test, but in situ carcinoma is increasing, which may be due to an increase of women being subjected to the risk factors.

What are the possible causes?

• Early age of first sexual intercourse
• Multiple partners
• Birth control pills
• Smoking
• Heavy metal and environmental toxicity
• Nutritional deficiencies
• Viral infections (especially herpes and human papilloma virus)
• Past trauma and/or abuse

For women with class 4 on the Pap smear test it is very important to first establish if the carcinoma is in situ, and therefore a biopsy is needed. A woman with recurrent class 3 Paps should also be biopsied, since she is at a higher risk, especially if many of the other risk factors are also present. It is of utmost importance to be under orthodox medical care. However, it is also important to look at improving the nutritional status of the body, improving the balance of the mind, healing past emotional traumas, and reducing all other known risk factors.

What are the psychosomatic causes?

In the psychosomatic context cancer may be the result of many years of negative thought patterns and beliefs, which slowly start to eat away at the self. Something traumatic may have happened in childhood, when we are open and vulnerable, which weakens the energy field around us. If left unresolved it can give rise to deep-seated fear, anger, sadness, grief, guilt and hopelessness, which if bottled up starts to affect our internal organs. Many women are frightened of their emotions, especially anger, and try desperately to cover it up by being 'nice' or blaming others for their own problems, thereby projecting their anger on to someone else.

Everyone carries cancer cells, but when we are strong and healthy our bodies reject them. They only start to accumulate and grow when we allow them to do so, by weakening our immune system. This can happen when we don't look after ourselves on the physical, emotional, mental and spiritual levels. If we abuse our bodies, carry resentment, anger, grief and sadness bottled up inside us, constantly engage in negative thinking, and feel a lack of purpose in life, it is easy to see how this can cause fertile ground for various illnesses to take hold.

Dysmenorrhoea (painful periods)

This is when painful cramps are experienced just before and during menstruation. It can also cause backache, bloating, abdominal pain and headache. It is not normal to experience cramps, and it is an indication that something is out of balance. It may be due to a variety of factors and it is important to establish the cause, so that appropriate treatment can be given. To just mask the symptoms by taking birth control pills is not desired, since this throws the body out of balance even further.

What causes it?

• Poor abdominal and pelvic floor muscle tone, leading to a 'drop' of pelvic organs, which can cause pelvic congestion and decreased circulation.
• Poor spinal mechanics leading to compromised nerve function to pelvic organs.
• Increased lumbar curvature, which can be genetic or caused by something as common as wearing high-heeled shoes. This can lead to a prolapse of the abdominal organs and decreased function of the spine, which can then affect the nerve supply to the pelvic organs.
• Lack of exercise, which leads to poor muscular support from the pelvic floor and abdomen
• Poor dietary habits, leading to nutritional deficiencies, especially B vitamins, calcium and iron. A heavy consumption of coffee, tea, cola, carbonated drinks, excess salt and meat can all result in these deficiencies, especially calcium.
• B vitamin deficiency, since these are needed for the breakdown of oestrogen in the liver.
• Methylxanthines in coffee, tea and cola have been linked to dysmenorrhoea and PMT.
• Liver congestion, which can be due to poor dietary and drinking habits, putting an increased stress on the liver

• Chronic constipation, since this allows for the re-absorption of waste products
• Dysfunction of the thyroid or the pituitary
• Low levels of progesterone, which can be due to an under-functioning thyroid
• Uterine overproduction of prostaglandins, since prostaglandins increase uterine contractions
• Endometriosis, pelvic inflammatory disease and ovarian cysts are other examples of pathology that can cause dysmenorrhoea.

What are the psychosomatic causes?

In a psychosomatic context dysmenorrhoea may indicate an individual who is feeling confused about becoming or being a woman. She may have deep feelings of guilt and/or repressed anger about her sexuality and about her ability to express love through her sexual energy. It may also be an indication that there is a deep inner longing for a child, and the pain felt during each menstruation is the emotional pain of realising that the longing for a child has yet again not been fulfilled.

Endometriosis

This is the second most common gynaecological disorder requiring hospital treatment and it is most commonly found in women over the age of thirty. It is a condition in which the cells lining the womb starts to grow outside of the uterus, such as in the ovaries, fallopian tubes, bladder and bowel. These cells still respond to the natural menstrual cycle and fill with blood each month, but there is nowhere for them to shed the blood. This can lead to inflammation and pain in the affected areas and development of fibrosis adhesions making organs stick together. If the endometriosis is extreme it can even lead to infertility, often due to the fallopian tubes becoming scarred.

What are the common symptoms?

• Painful ovulation
• Painful periods
• Painful intercourse
• Bloating
• Back pain
• Heavy and irregular bleeding
• Tiredness

What causes it?

There is no known cause of this condition, but there are a few possible theories, such as:
• Early onset of menstruation, which means that more menstrual cycles occur before a pregnancy
• Reflux menstruation, which is when menstrual blood backs up into the fallopian tubes and enters the pelvic cavity
• Increased oestrogen production
• Long-term treatment of antibiotics or steroids, which can lead to malabsorption due to a sharp decrease in healthy gut flora
• Immune system damage caused by the environmental pollutant dioxin. According to research done by the U.S. Endometriosis Protection Agency there seems to be a link between dioxin levels in the body and increased risk and severity of endometriosis. Dioxin is a bi-product of chlorine, which is used in plastic, drugs, dry-cleaning fluid, disinfectants, pesticides and wood preservatives. When it is being burnt it becomes airborne and then falls on plants and grass, which is then eaten by animals, such as cows. It then enters the human food chain, and is especially prevalent in meat and dairy products.
• Poor posture and spinal function, which can lead to a disturbance in the nerve, blood and lymphatic flow to the pelvic organs.
• Past trauma and abuse

What are the psychosomatic causes?

In a psychosomatic context endometriosis may be an indication of an individual who is having a deep inner conflict relating to being a woman, a mother, and/or a lover. Perhaps there is deep guilt or maybe she feels betrayed.

It may also be an indication of an intense longing for a child, for someone to nurture or even for a chance to give birth to the inner self. When this longing is unfulfilled the inner lining of the womb starts to expand into nearby areas in a desperate attempt to fulfill this wish.

Fibroids

This is a non-malignant growth in the uterus. It usually gives no symptoms, but it may give painful heavy periods, bleeding between periods, and if fairly large can give a feeling of pressure in the abdomen.

What causes it?

• An excess of oestrogen in the body, such as from the pill or HRT
• Poor nutrition
• Constipation
• Liver dysfunction
• Other hormonal imbalances
• Unresolved issues relating to past trauma and/or abuse

What are the psychosomatic causes?

In a psychosomatic context fibroids may indicate deeply suppressed negative thought patterns, relating to our femininity, our sexuality or our role as a mother. This may relate to any past trauma, abuse or guilt we have experienced due to us being female.

Menopause

Menopause is a natural occurrence in the body, probably intended to relieve a woman from the strain of bearing children when she reaches a mature age of around 50.

What causes a natural menopause?

It is due to a gradual process of decreased oestrogen output by the ovaries, and in a healthy individual it should bring very few, if any, side effects.

What can bring on an unnatural menopause?

Thyroid malfunction, liver dysfunction and removal of uterus and/or ovaries. The latter causes the most severe form of menopause, and if this affects a woman before the normal onset of menopause, HRT may be indicated.

What happens in the body when the ovaries reduce their production of oestrogens?

The pituitary sends out signals to other glands to take over. This is especially so for the adrenal glands; however, if they are exhausted due to poor nutrition, diet deficiencies, stress and/or hypoglycaemia, then this back-up system fails, and may lead to menopausal symptoms.

What are the common symptoms?

Cold sweats, hot flashes, headaches, depression, palpitation, cold hands and feet, urinary tract infections, forgetfulness, lack of concentration, loss of libido and dry vagina.

What can worsen menopausal symptoms?

A food intolerance can worsen symptoms. There is a higher occurrence of this around the time of menopause, which may be due to increased build-up of toxins over the years, which now cannot be released through the menstrual flow; a decrease in the immune system; and adrenal exhaustion as the body and mind are trying to cope with the changes.

What about any psychological causes?

There is a direct link between how women react to menopause and how the society they live in views older women. In cultures where entering menopause is seen as a sign of developing wisdom and the woman earns greater respect from her peers, very few of the common side effects of menopause occur. These women tend to go through menopause without vaginitis, hot flashes and osteoporosis (3). This may partly be due to a better, more wholesome diet, but mostly to the psychological aspects of this positive attitude to menopause. In the western world beauty and youth are highly regarded, whilst getting older is seen as something negative and not worth much respect. Is there any wonder that many women dread stepping into this new phase of their lives, since it doesn't bring increased respect from the society around them? Maybe the real treatment lies in changing society's view on ageing.

What are the psychosomatic causes?

Entering menopause is a signal to ourselves that we are changing, that we are leaving behind a phase to enter into a new dimension of our lives. When we feel confused about our self-worth we may feel that our value is coming from how youthful, attractive, sexy and fertile we are. We then feel sad, depressed and anxious about this change, because we worry whether we will still be loved, cherished and wanted. So instead of embracing menopause, we resent it, which creates enormous inner tension.

Ovarian cysts

These are fluid-filled tumours of the ovary, which usually give rise to no symptoms. For some it can lead to a sudden onset of pain that can be felt on one side of the abdomen at the time of ovulation, which usually occurs half way between menstrual cycles.

What causes it?

- Poor diet leading to nutritional deficiencies
- Gastro-intestinal dysfunction
- Toxic bowel and liver
- Hormone and/or endocrine imbalance
- Spinal dysfunctions leading to inadequate nerve, blood and lymphatic supply to the pelvic organs
- Past abuse/trauma

What are the psychosomatic causes?

In a psychosomatic context ovaries are the seat of a woman's feminine creative energy, so an ovarian cyst may be an indication of a woman who is experiencing blocked emotional energy relating to all aspects of her being a woman. Perhaps there is an inner conflict relating to her femininity, or with being a mother. Maybe there has been unhealed past abuse, and the repressed emotional energy from that is starting to take on physical form. It can also be an indication that she is trying to give birth to a new self, but an inner conflict is holding her back. However, the longing for this new self is still there, so her unconscious mind starts to create a cyst as a symbol of this inner yearning.

Pre-menstrual Tension Syndrome (PMS)

This is a cyclical syndrome related to the menstrual cycle giving rise to a variety of symptoms usually 4–14 days before menstruation.

What are the symptoms?

Mood swings, irritability, personality changes, depression, anxiety, crying, cravings for sweets, breast tenderness, bloating, acne, headaches and back pain. The symptoms usually end at the onset of the period.

What are the causes?

There is no doubt that PMS is caused by hormonal changes related to the menstrual cycle, but what makes some women more prone than others?

It has been found that women with PMS tend to eat more refined carbohydrates, refined sugar, more salt and more dairy.

They tend to be deficient in zinc, manganese, magnesium, iron and B6.

Stress leads to a lack of vitamin C, since this is used to buffer the increased release of adrenaline from the adrenal glands (initial response to stress). Stress also affects the hypothalamus, which in turn affects the pituitary, ovaries and adrenal glands. This in itself can change the hormone levels in the body. Also adrenal exhaustion can lead to a deficiency in oestrogen, since the adrenals are responsible for about 20% of oestrogen production in the body. Prolonged periods of stress can also lead to dopamine deficiency, which has been linked to some types of PMS.

Another cause is hypoglycaemia (low blood sugar), which occurs when the diet is rich in refined carbohydrates, sugar, sweets, biscuits, coffee and alcohol. Hypoglycaemia itself does not cause PMS, since it is a response to food, but it overburdens the adrenal glands as they try to cope with the blood sugar fluctuations.

High caffeine consumption leads to an overuse of the adrenal glands.

Refined carbohydrates are stripped of their B content (such as white bread, white pasta and white rice), and the adrenal glands need both B-vitamins and vitamin C to function. Therefore stress and poor diet lead to a shortage of B-complex, especially B6, and vitamin C in the body.

Many women suffering with PMS have also been shown to have a low thyroid function. Therefore, it is important to have the thyroid examined.

Lead poisoning can lead to PMS, since it interferes with oestrogen's binding capacity, and can cause hormonal changes.

It also seems that some PMS sufferers have not developed good coping techniques, thereby increasing the stress levels of everyday life.

What are the psychosomatic causes?

In a psychosomatic context PMS may be an indication of a woman who feels inner emotional and mental confusion about herself, her life, her femininity, her relationships, motherhood and/or her work. This creates inner tension, which she may be able to deal with on the surface relatively well until her hormones start to fluctuate with her monthly cycle. As her body prepares to shed the unwanted waste products, her unconscious mind then takes the opportunity to release repressed negative emotions as well. This allows the woman to get in contact with her deep emotional side, and to let go of past emotional and mental pain and confusion regularly.

Advice for all conditions

How can I help in regards to my diet?

• Eat small, frequent meals to decrease stress on the pancreas and adrenal glands.

• Eat plenty of fruits and vegetables, seeds, nuts, beans, legumes, whole grains, soya, and fish. This will increase the fibre content, which will help bind to oestrogen in the gut and reduce the oestrogen content in the body.

• Eat wholemeal bread, brown rice and brown pasta.

• Eat lots of soya products, because they contain phyto-oestrogens.

• Sprinkle wheatgerm on food every day. It is very high in iron, essential fatty acids and B-vitamins.

• Drink diluted freshly juiced carrots, beetroot and lemon daily to cleanse and nourish the kidneys and liver.

• Ensure healthy functioning of the bowel by taking whole linseeds daily and a spoon of olive oil.

What should I avoid?

• Avoid all red meat, since it has a very high oestrogen content which increases the risk of developing most of these conditions, especially cervical dysplasia.

• Avoid all sugar, honey, pure fruit juices (instead dilute with water), soft drinks, sweets, cakes, biscuits, white bread, white pasta and white rice. These are all refined carbohydrates and will convert to glucose too quickly in the blood stream giving rise to hypoglycaemia and contributing to adrenal exhaustion.

• Decrease intake of all dairy products (except for organic live yoghurt).

• Avoid smoking and alcohol.

• Until chlorine use is reduced the only way to decrease dioxin ingestion is by cutting out all animal fat, meat and dairy products (endometriosis).

• Avoid all caffeine, such as in coffee, cola and chocolate.

• Some medications can aggravate these conditions, such as birth control pills (oestrogen increases risk of cervical dysplasia and endometriosis) and asthma medications (caffeine increases risk of endometriosis). See your medical doctor for advice.

Which supplements and herbs help?

• A good multivitamin and mineral complex.

• Vitamin C with bioflavonoids is important to alleviate the burden on the adrenal glands, as well as help the efficiency of the insulin. It also acts as a weak blocker of the body's oestrogen receptors, so is useful in cervical dysplasia, endometriosis, fibroids and ovarian cysts.

• B-complex is needed for proper function of carbohydrate metabolism, as well as for the function of the adrenal glands.

• Extra supplementation with B6 has shown to be very helpful (PMS, dysmenorrhea, cervical dysplasia). Antioxidants (A, C and E) are also often useful.

• Zinc is often deficient in women with menopausal symptoms. It is also needed for insulin production as well as helping to combat the side effects of stress, thereby improving the immune system.

• For cervical dysplasia take extra selenium, since this has been shown to be low. Also take zinc to boost immune system.

• Magnesium (preferably combined with calcium) is important in the control of blood sugar levels and can also help to alleviate menstrual cramps.

• Spirulina is very useful to help normalise blood glucose levels.

• Evening primrose oil and flaxseed oil taken daily are useful for balancing the hormones.

They also contain vitamin E, which helps to alleviate dry vagina during menopause.
• Aloe vera juice, royal jelly and wild yam are useful during menopause.
• Lactobacillus acidophilus capsules to improve intestinal function and to reduce the re-absorption of excreted oestrogens.
• Various herbs may be of help, such as liquorice for lowering oestrogen levels, valerian and dong quai for menstrual cramps, chaste berry for painful breasts, black cohosh and dong quai for hot flashes and gingko biloba for improving circulation and memory.

How else can I improve my physical health?

• Avoid taking the birth control pill.
• Avoid using make-up, skin and hair products with chemicals; instead use organic, natural alternatives.
• Regular hot and cold sitz baths increase circulation to the pelvic organs
• Castor oil packs to the liver and over the affected areas weekly.
• Exercise helps to improve circulation, improve heart function, improve ability to cope with stress, improve oxygen to all tissues (including brain, which helps to improve memory), improve energy levels, decrease bone loss, decrease cholesterol levels and reduce blood pressure.

How can I improve my emotional, mental and spiritual health?

Daily breathing exercises and meditation.

Find out your values for being a woman. (see Chapter One, values in coaching programme). Do you have any limiting beliefs which have formed any away from values?

What does the ideal YOU look like? What qualities does she have? Trace back to the qualities she would have and then feel, see and hear your-self being these qualities, acting from these qualities. Notice in which ways you are different, and ask your unconscious mind which steps you need to take to achieve being your ideal self.

The key to release a negative emotion is to feel it fully so that you know it is there, and then to find out what it wants to communicate to you, what positive teaching it is bringing you. If you feel it but put a lock on it by either refusing to accept it, or keep yourself so busy that you cannot possibly acknowledge it, it has no other choice but to go deep within your unconscious mind. In doing so it will follow you wherever you go, and will keep drawing situations to you, which mirror why you experienced the negative emotion in the first place. When you release your negative emotions from the past you free yourself to fully experience life in the present moment.

With the aid of the coaching programme release all negative emotions, limiting beliefs, past traumatic events, emotional pain caused by unwanted states and behaviours held in the body, and do the forgiveness exercise with all your relationships as well as your condition.

What is it within you that you would like to give birth to? In which ways can you allow your own inner beauty and light to shine forth into the world? Think deeply about these questions, because the answers hold the truth about your purpose for being here and reveal to you your authentic self.

Meditate on your condition. Send it as much love as you possibly can.

A good meditation to do regularly is the following: sit comfortably with your feet on the ground. Open up the soles of your feet and visualise all your anger draining away from your spirit, mind and body through the soles of your feet and collecting into a ball on the ground. Then visualise how you place this ball of anger on a fire, and see how the blue-white heat from the fire purifies the anger until it is all gone. Then up from the fire a new positive emotion is rising, which is a gift to you. Breathe in this positive emotion. Let it fill your lungs, and as you breathe out let it flow to every cell of your being—body, mind and spirit. Now do the same for all your other negative emotions.

Practice seeing the positive in every situation in your life. There is always a positive lesson waiting to be discovered even in the most traumatic experience.

Allow yourself to live your life the way that brings you the most happiness.

Additional advice for menopause:

Cherish this new phase in your life. Look at everything you have learnt. Isn't it true that you are able to look at yourself and life with more wisdom than you did twenty years ago? Aren't these qualities wonderful gifts to share with others?

Develop a relaxed attitude about getting older. View it in a positive light. Do the forgiveness exercise with the part of you that wants to remain young.

See life from a larger perspective. Notice how much you have grown during your life, from birth up until now, and envision how much you will continue to grow. See all the love you have given and received, all the positive experiences you have had and the amazing life lessons you have encountered, and feel how much wisdom you have gained as you have grown older. Your body has been an amazing vehicle which has allowed you to experience all this.

Which therapies help?

Tibetan, ayurvedic and Chinese medicine help to balance the hormones and the nervous system, aiding the body to heal.

Osteopathy, cranial osteopathy and chiropractic help to improve the blood flow to the pelvic organs and to balance the nervous system.

Medical herbalism and homeopathy help improve the hormone balance and immune system.

Yoga (Triangle, Spinal Twist and the Bow) and **Pilates** (Spinal Twist and the Mermaid) exercises help improve nerve and blood supply to all the pelvic organs. Avoid all inverted postures (upside down) when menstruating.

Healing helps by restoring energy as well as balancing the emotions.

NLP, hypnotherapy and well-being coaching help by releasing past negative emotions and limiting beliefs.

Useful affirmations

I am a beautiful woman filled with strength, power and wisdom. I create my own life and my own reality."

"I let go of the past with love, and embrace the new with love and joy."

"I now forgive everyone who I perceive has hurt me in the past. As I forgive them I set myself free."

Common Gastro-Intestinal Conditions

The following conditions are covered together, because the treatments are usually very similar.

Gastritis

This is a condition where the mucous membrane lining the stomach is inflamed. It gives pain over the upper abdomen and the stomach may be distended. It can also give nausea, vomiting and diarrhoea.

What are the causes?

- Overeating
- Poor diet (refined carbohydrates, fried, spicy and salty food)
- Improper food combining
- Large intake of alcohol
- Smoking
- Caffeine
- Stress, both emotional and physical, such as from flu, major surgery or severe burns
- Various medications (aspirin, ibuprofen and steroids)
- Food allergies/sensitivities
- Unbalanced production of hydrochloric acid (HCI)
- Helicobacter pylori infection
- Viral infection

Atrophic gastritis is found particularly in the elderly, where the body destroys the digestive tract lining. This can lead to B12 deficiency resulting in pernicious anaemia.

What about the psychosomatic causes?

Gastritis may point to something in our environment that we have to absorb or deal with which is irritating us, causing our very organ of assimilation to become inflamed with frustration, anxiety or anger in having to process it.

Heartburn

This condition is felt as a burning sensation in the stomach and over the chest area, which may radiate into the neck if stomach acid is regurgitating into the throat, giving an acidic reflux into the mouth.

What causes it?

- Obesity
- Pregnancy
- Poor posture causing compression over the anterior ribcage, compromising the function of the stomach. If restrictions within the thoracic spine are also present the nerve and blood supply to the digestive tract may be impaired.
- Eating too much at mealtime, especially fried, spicy or fatty foods, tomato-based foods, citrus fruits, coffee, alcohol, chocolate, and carbonated drinks
- Drinking liquid with meals, since this dilutes the digestive enzymes
- Eating quickly, especially if late at night, or if stressed
- Stress and anxiety
- Common dysfunctions, such as ulcers and hiatus hernia, ileo-caecal valve problems, gall-bladder problems, low levels of digestive enzymes and abnormal hydrochloric acid levels and food allergies/sensitivities
- Cigarette smoking
- Helicobacter pylori, Epstein-Barr virus and candida albicans

What are the psychosomatic causes?

Heartburn and heart disease have similar causes,

such as problems relating to how we deal with the emotional aspects of ourselves. It may indicate lack of joy in our life, stress, emotional instability, insecurity and a burning fear of life and what it may bring. It may also be due to an inability to stand up for oneself, establish boundaries and being able to say no. This leads to increased internal tension, which places a heavy burden on the heart. It may also indicate a person who places far too much value on things, which give little lasting joy, such as money, power and status.

Hiatus hernia

This is a common condition where the stomach protrudes through the oesophageal opening in the diaphragm. This leads to a reflux regurgitation of stomach acid, which can lead to heartburn, discomfort when lying down, pain behind the sternum, swallowing difficulties, inflammation and ulceration.

What are the possible causes?

• Pregnancy, obesity, constipation and heavy lifting, which increase the intra-abdominal pressure
• Vitamin and mineral deficiencies leading to a weakening of the nearby tissues
• Over-consumption of spicy food
• Digestive and ileo-caecal valve problems
• Smoking
• Spinal dysfunctions
• Weakened diaphragm
• Poor abdominal tone and poor posture
• Previous trauma to the area

What are the psychosomatic causes?

A hernia may represent a rupture in a relationship, with ourselves or another person. When the hernia is affecting the stomach it may indicate that something in our near environment, which we need to assimilate and digest, is causing us strain and pressure. There is a conflict between our external world (outside pressure) and our internal world (stomach).

Indigestion

Indigestion is also referred to as dyspepsia and acid stomach, and it is characterised by a discomfort in the upper abdomen. It is always a sign that the digestive tract is not functioning properly.

What are the common causes?

Depending on the timing of the symptoms different causes are possible. If there is pain on eating it may indicate esophagitis, gastritis or a gastric (stomach) ulcer. If there is pain 45–60 minutes after eating or during the night it may indicate a duodenal ulcer (see **Ulcers**). Indigestion can also give severe chest pain very similar to angina, and a heart attack may sometimes give pain similar to indigestion (especially in women); therefore, pain in upper abdomen should always be investigated.

Other possible causes of indigestion:
• Eating quickly and not chewing properly
• Stress and emotional upsets
• Eating while under stress
• Eating too much when ill. Children and animals will never eat when ill, because the body is busy dealing with the immune support and it does not need the added pressure of dealing with food substances. Liquids and fruits are allowed. (See **Colds, Flu and Sinusitis**)
• Excess of acid-forming foods, such as refined carbohydrates and sugar
• Excess of saturated animal fat in the diet
• Digestive enzyme deficiency
• Food allergies, most commonly milk and wheat
• Strong spices and salt
• Low fibre diet

• Excess of tea, coffee or alcohol
• Eating fruit after a meal and eating unripe fruit, which is high in pectin, making it difficult to digest
• Spinal dysfunctions (neck, thoracic and ribs) causing decreased nerve and blood supply to the gastro-intestinal tract
• Poor posture leading to increased strain and pressure on the digestive tract

What are the psychosomatic causes?

In a psychosomatic context indigestion may be an indication that something or someone in our life is difficult to digest. Perhaps a situation or a relationship is causing us anxiety, anger or extreme stress; we react against it and are unwilling to assimilate it, hence the indigestion.

Inflammatory Bowel Disease (IBD)

This consists of two disorders—Crohn's disease and ulcerative colitis—which usually occur between the ages of 15–35. They share many common features and have both been linked to an increased risk of colon cancer.

What is Crohn's disease?

Crohn's disease is a non-specific, chronic inflammation of the intestinal wall, which can affect any part of the gastrointestinal tract (mouth to anus), but mainly affects the ileum and the terminal portion of the small intestines. It gives a variety of symptoms, such as abdominal pain over the affected area (usually the right lower abdomen), diarrhoea, weight-loss, low-grade fever, tiredness, skin problems and joint pain.

What is ulcerative colitis?

This is a chronic, non-specific inflammatory condition involving the lining of the colon where small ulcers and abscesses are formed. The symptoms are very similar to those in Crohn's with the difference that the diarrhoea is bloody and the patient will experience painful cramps in the lower part of the abdomen. There may also be haemorrhoids, fissures, fistulas and abscesses in the rectum.

What are the causes?

There is a genetic tendency to IBD in Jews and Caucasians; 15–40% of cases are hereditary.

Diet plays a role, with the typical western diet being the worst offender. IBD is uncommon in countries with a primitive diet, but on the increase in western societies. Studies have shown that people who develop Crohn's have a diet high in saturated fat, refined carbohydrates, and sugar, whilst low in fruit and vegetables (6,7). It also may be linked with food allergies.

Others seem to have found a controversial link between developing Crohn's disease and the measles/mumps/rubella (MMR) vaccine.

Some theories suggest IBD may be linked to a previous infection by a virus, bacteria, fungus or parasite.

Another theory suggests it may be linked with antibiotic use, where antibiotics have been administered improperly (not the correct dose or type); therefore, the good, healthy intestinal flora is wiped out, whilst the infectious agent remains and can multiply (and produce toxins) to become even more resistant to the antibiotics (8).

IBD seems to cause an abnormal immune response or it may be linked with autoimmune disorders.

Emotional stress may also cause or aggravate IBD.

What are the psychosomatic causes?

In a psychosomatic context inflammation may indicate inflamed anger, or deeply buried emotions that need to be let out. When it occurs in our intestines—the very place where we integrate our outer reality with our inner world, decide what is nourishing us, and what we need to get rid of—it may indicate a conflict between what we need to release from the past and get out of our system and our unwillingness to do so. It may be that we are afraid of feeling the emotions (anger, fear, sadness) that are connected with the issues that need to be released; instead we hold onto them, trying to bury them in our bodies, where they cause inflammation and pain.

Irritable Bowel Syndrome (IBS)

This is a common condition in which the large intestine fails to function properly.

What are the most common symptoms?

The most common symptoms are abdominal pain and bloating, which is relieved by bowel movements, although there may still be a feeling of incomplete emptying. Other symptoms include constipation, diarrhoea, flatulence, excess mucus secretion in stools, nausea, depression, anxiety, weight fluctuations, back pain, neck pain and teeth grinding.

What are the causes?

IBS can be caused by food allergies, antibiotics, laxative abuse, depression, anxiety, stress, fatigue, low fibre diet and other dietary factors.

What are the psychosomatic causes?

Any problem with the bowels indicates that we may have an inability to let go of the past and allow ourselves to digest and assimilate our present life and reality. Perhaps we are refusing to forgive others for events we perceive as painful and unacceptable, so we literally shut down our inner function, causing constipation. Or we try to run away from issues, which causes inner stress and speeds up our bowels, leading to diarrhoea. Both types of behaviour lead to enormous inner stress and conflict and IBS only mirrors that.

Peptic Ulcer

This is an erosion of the mucous membrane either in the stomach or the duodenum.

What are the symptoms?

If the ulcer is in the duodenum, pain comes on 2–4 hours after eating, is aggravated by hunger, coffee or alcohol, and relieved by food. The patient usually wakes up in the early hours of the morning with stomach pain. If the ulcer is in the stomach (gastric), pain is experienced just after eating.

What causes it?

The main cause is probably a helicobacter pylori infection, which initiates a secretion of an enzyme that leads to an erosion of the mucosal lining of the stomach or duodenum. The helicobacter pylori bacteria is found in 70–75% of patients with gastric ulcers and 90–100% of patients with duodenal ulcers.

Other causes may be:
• Food allergies. Some studies have shown a link between peptic ulcer and allergies (4).
• High consumption of coffee, tea, tobacco,

alcohol, spicy or fried food, which all increase acid secretion
• A low fibre diet, since a diet rich in fibre is associated with a low rate of duodenal ulcers
• Smoking
• Stress
• Medications, such as aspirin, anti-inflammatories, steroids and antacids (the latter due to a rebound effect)

A link has also been established between blood group O and increased risk of stomach ulcers, possibly due to the high acid content in type O individuals (5).

From an osteopathic and chiropractic point of view, spinal restriction between thoracic vertebrae 4 and thoracic 9, as well as occiput/cervical 1, can aggravate and accelerate an imbalance in the digestive process, since the nerve flow to stomach and intestines comes from these segments. This in turn can affect the blood flow to these organs, which can impair their function.

What are the psychosomatic causes?

An ulcer may be an indication of an individual who is bottling up intense emotions, such as anger, irritation, anxiety or fear, which start to eat away at the self. The stomach is the area where we take in our experiences and digest them to make them nourishing for us. If we find that someone or something in our reality is causing us to feel fear, anger or irritation, but we cannot show it outwardly or deal with it appropriately, it may start to upset our stomach, causing intense pain. It may also indicate a person who believes he is not good enough, so he is not allowing himself to get nourished from his outside environment.

Advice for all conditions

How can I help in regards to my diet?

• Always chew food properly and eat small, frequent meals.
• Eat only when relaxed and always sit down for a meal.
• Drink plenty of water every day.
• Drink herbal teas and dandelion coffee.
• Eat oily fish, chicken, tofu and soya, except if soya intolerant.
• Increase dietary fibres—preferably from vegetables, fruits, brown rice, seeds (especially linseeds), legumes and pulses. Be careful with large amounts of bran, since too much can have a negative effect on the digestive system. If more fibre is needed than can be acquired from the foods listed above, supplement with small amounts of psyllium husks or seeds.
• Instead of wheat, eat rye bread, rice cakes or oat biscuits.
• If both dairy and soya intolerance are present, oat or rice milk are excellent substitutes.
• One litre of cabbage juice per day is excellent in the treatment for most gastro-intestinal conditions, especially peptic ulcers. It contains an anti-ulcer vitamin, vitamin U. If needed take cabbage extract, Cabagin/vitamin U.
• Food combining may be highly beneficial. This means not to mix protein (fish, meat, chicken) and carbohydrates (rice, pasta, bread) at the same meal. Protein needs an acid environment, whilst carbohydrates need a neutral environment. Therefore by eating them at separate times less strain is put on the stomach. Eat either proteins or carbohydrates with vegetables.
• For hiatus hernia it is important to change the diet to improve proper bowel function (see Constipation).

What should I avoid?

• Cut out spicy foods, sugar, salt, red meat, citrus fruits, nuts and food additives.

• Eliminate food sensitivities—the most common ones being dairy, corn, wheat, yeast, beef and pork. Studies have shown a link between IBS and food allergies/sensitivities (9,10,11). Avoid wheat in bran, biscuits, cakes, and breakfast cereals. Some people can tolerate wheat in pasta, but it is better avoided to start with and then reintroduced slowly to see if the body is able to cope with it.

• Avoid fried, salty and fatty foods, alcohol, milk, coffee and tea, since they all increase stomach acid secretion.

• Avoid all refined carbohydrates since they increase the production of stomach acid.

• Do not combine fruits (especially citrus) and starches (such as cereals).

• Avoid fruits with small seeds, such as raspberries and strawberries, because they can irritate the gut lining.

• Avoid tobacco, aspirin and NSAIDs.

• Never drink with meals. Instead drink 20 minutes before eating or 30 minutes after.

• Do not eat very large meals.

• Never eat when stressed or angry.

• Do not sit slouched during and after a meal, since this puts added pressure on the stomach.

• Do not wear tight fitting clothes or belts.

• For hiatus hernia avoid heavy lifting.

Which supplements and herbs help?

• If you have a viral infection improve your immune system (see **Immune System**).

• Take a few tablespoons of whole linseeds daily to aid proper bowel function.

• Vitamin C with bioflavonoids aids tissue repair.

• B-complex helps calm the nervous system.

• Vitamins A and E, zinc and selenium are useful.

• Fish oil and flax seed oil help to decrease an inflammatory response (IBD and gastritis).

• Cinnamon and ginger help digestion.

• Lactobacillus acidophilus capsules help the healthy functioning of the intestinal flora.

• Deglycyrrhizinated liquorice (DGL) may be helpful in the treatment of ulcers and gastritis.

• Aloe vera, slippery elm, marshmallow and cabbage juice are all very good for soothing and healing the lining of the stomach and intestines.

• Quercetin is useful as an anti-inflammatory in IBD.

• Check if helicobacter pylori infection is present. If it is, a course of antibiotics may be necessary, in which case it will be necessary to take extra lactobacillus acidophilus.

How else can I improve my physical health?

Regular hot and cold packs to the area between your shoulder blades and upper neck will stimulate your circulation there, which will aid your nerve supply to the gut.

Get regular exercise. This allows excess adrenaline from stress to be used up, and your brain will have a chance to release endorphins, which are natural mood enhancers. This aids relaxation, which is beneficial for your digestive system.

How can I improve my emotional, mental and spiritual health?

Learn to let go of negative emotions. Whenever you harbour anger, frustration or irritation you only hurt yourself. So let it go.

With the coaching programme release negative emotions, limiting beliefs, pain held in the body and do the forgiveness exercise.

Look for the wisdom in any situation in your life. This allows you to un-hook all the negative emotions from your mind, so that you are left with love, joy and compassion. This will have a massive positive impact on your health.

If you find yourself complaining about your health or a particular person in your life, stop! Gently send that thought away, and replace it with something positive and nurturing.

If something is irritating you in your environment, look for the real problem, and see what steps you can take to improve it. If it is your work environment, perhaps it is time for you to either change your work, or change your perception about it. If it is someone you know, try to see the situation through her eyes. How would you feel if you were in her place? Do the forgiveness exercise in regards to this person. Once you have done this, you should have a better idea of how to solve the problem. Sometimes all we need to do is give up our attachment to having a person be the way we want her to be, and see her for who she truly is.

Start establishing your boundaries, both in your professional and personal lives. Only you can initiate the change. Look at what is causing you the most stress, and see what you can do to change it. The solution is always present in the problem itself, so look for it. Perhaps you need to delegate some of your tasks and responsibilities. Or maybe you are allowing someone to abuse you. Perhaps they abuse your trust or goodwill, or they know that you never oppose their demands or bad behaviour. Maybe you put everyone else first, and never allow yourself some rest. Whatever it is, look at it and then do something about it.

Look at all the tasks you have to do in a week. Most of us take on far too much, because we are afraid that if we say no to others, they will not like us. Make a list of all your tasks for the whole week, and then prioritise them on a scale from 1–5 in order of importance, with 1 being not important and 5 being highly important. Now make another list, and this time write down

only the tasks that got a 4 or a 5. How much has this cut down your list? How much time have you just freed up if you were to let go of all the others tasks? What could you do with this time, which could benefit your inner well-being?

Practice meditation daily.

Here is a good visualization: Sit in a comfortable position and allow yourself to sink into the inner stillness. If you find that your mind is frantic, practice some breathing exercises for a few minutes (breathe in slowly through your nose and out slowly through your mouth). Once you find the stillness, visualise drawing light to yourself. Let this light enter through the top or your head and let it flow down your neck and spine. Feel your brain and spine become balanced and energised, and then see how this light flows from your spine through all the little nerves into your stomach and intestines. Feel how this light soothes and heals the lining and all the tissues of your digestive tract. Send your condition as much love as you possibly can.

Ask your digestive tract what it wants you to pay attention to, know or learn, which would help it heal. Then act on this guidance.

At the end of each day tell yourself or someone you love three good things that have happened to you that day. This trains your mind to look for the positives in life, and remember that you get what you focus on, so focus on wonderful things.

Which therapies help?

Tibetan, ayurvedic and Chinese medicine help by improving the function of the digestive tract, spine, adrenal glands, liver and nervous system.

Reflexology, shiatzu and acupressure help by stimulating pressure points relating to the digestive system, thoracic spine, adrenal glands and liver.

Osteopathy and chiropractic help by improving function of the digestive tract. Visceral techniques help to reduce tension within the fascia surrounding the gut, which improves tissue health. Cranial osteopathy also helps to balance the nervous system.

Pilates and yoga help by balancing your neuro-musculo-skeletal system. Specific exercises, such as the Spinal Twist and Pelvic Bridging are useful for improving the spinal function for the specific areas which deal with the digestive tract. It is important to avoid inverted postures (may aggravate inflamed gastro-intestinal structures) or postures increasing compression of the neck (irritates the vagus nerve supplying the gut), such as the Cobra.

Healing helps by releasing negative emotions from the unconscious mind (the body) without engaging the conscious mind.

Kinesiology helps by addressing any underlying food allergies or sensitivities.

NLP, hypnotherapy and well-being coaching help by releasing negative emotions, limiting beliefs and setting up more positive coping strategies.

Useful affirmations

"My heart is filled with love and joy and I share this love and joy with others."

"It is now safe for me to fully experience everything in my life."

"I now let go of the old and embrace the new."

"My thoughts are filled with love and compassion."

Constipation

This condition is present when you are unable to have daily bowel movements or have pain during bowel movements.

What is it caused by?

• Not drinking enough water and not eating enough food with a high water content
• Drinking too much black tea
• Too little fibre in the diet
• Not enough cardiovascular exercise
• Stress, since this activates the sympathetic nervous system, which effectively shuts down digestive function
• Eating disorders and laxative abuse
• Bowel disease
• Pregnancy
• Spinal restrictions affecting the nerves to the digestive tract
• Side effects of various drugs, such as painkillers and blood pressure tablets
• Food sensitivities and allergies
• Iron supplements

What are the psychosomatic causes?

In a psychosomatic context constipation may be indicative of refusing to let go of the past, of trying to control our environment and experiences by holding onto them for fear of letting go. There may be difficulty with 'going with the flow' and an inability to relax and just allow life to be as it is.

How can I help in regards to my diet?

• Drink plenty of water and eat lots of fruits and vegetables with a high water content.
• Increase fibre in your diet, and eat plenty of dried fruits. Make sure to also drink adequately,

otherwise the increased consumption of fibre will have a constipating effect.

What should I avoid?

Avoid dairy products, black tea and refined foods. Even though coffee has a diuretic and laxative effect, it is best to avoid it, since it upsets the natural workings of the gut.

How can I improve my physical health?

• Massage your abdomen for 5–10 minutes. Start massaging with small, circular movements at the lower left hand corner of the abdomen for a few minutes. This is because there will be some faeces here, waiting to come out, and this needs to be loosened first. Then go to the bottom right hand corner and work your way up to the ribcage, massage across the stomach, just under the ribs and then down on the left hand side.
• Exercise regularly, such as walking.
• Various yoga and Pilates exercises are highly beneficial, such as the Spinal Twist, Pelvic Bridging and the Sun Salutation.

Which supplements and herbs may help?

• Olive oil helps to soften the stools.
• An effective yet gentle laxative is to mix dried fruits with water, simmer for 15–30 minutes, until fruit is very soft. Drink one cup of this per day.
• B-complex supplementation may help, since folic acid deficiency may present with constipation.
• Take flax seed oil, aloe vera juice and lactobacillus acidophilus daily.
• Peppermint and caraway teas are beneficial.
• Psyllium husks and psyllium seeds mixed with water or juice may help as filling agents. If still no effect, then senna leaves may be used.

How can I improve my emotional, mental and spiritual health?

Practice meditation regularly, since this will balance your central nervous system and therefore aid your digestion.

Learn to let go of the past and embrace the now.

Sit down with your legs tucked up beneath you. Then start to fully relax your whole abdomen. Close your eyes and with your inner awareness travel around your intestines silently telling them to relax and let go of all the tension and all that they do not need. Do this for 5–10 minutes.

Another good visualisation is the following: Sit comfortably, with your spine erect. Focus on your breathing for a few minutes, and feel all the tension leave your mind and body. Then visualise the soles of your feet opening up and let all your tension and everything that you do not need drain away from your mind and body through the soles of your feet. As it enters the earth, it is transformed into positive energy. Keep letting go of everything you do not need, just keep sending it out of your mind and body through the soles of your feet. When you feel thoroughly cleansed, close the soles of your feet and then visualise opening up the top of your head. Draw in universal love energy through the top of your head and let it flow through your mind and body totally revitalising every cell of your being. Do this until you feel energised and refreshed.

Which therapies help?

Tibetan, ayurvedic and Chinese medicine and acupuncture help by assisting the digestive tract and promoting proper elimination.

Reflexology, acupressure and shiatzu help by stimulating pressure points, which aid bowel movements.

Osteopathy and chiropractic help by addressing structural problems, which are causing unnecessary strain and stress on the bowels, as well as helping to balance the nerve and blood supply to the gastro-intestinal tract. Cranial osteopathy helps especially in the treatment of children.

Kinesiology helps by establishing if there is an underlying food allergy/sensitivity present, which is upsetting the intestinal function.

Healing helps by balancing the emotions and releasing blocked energy.

Homeopathy has various remedies, which are useful for constipation, such as causticum (when stool is difficult to pass), nux vomica (when the sufferer is of an impatient and stressed nature) and silica (when there is lots of straining but no emptying of bowels).

Useful affirmations

"It is now safe for me to let go of the old and embrace the new."

"The changes of life are exciting and fulfilling."

"By allowing life to flow freely through me, my life is exciting and fulfilling."

Depression

Most of us have felt depressed at one point or another in our lives. For most, this passes after a short time, but for some this feeling of sadness lingers on, colouring every aspect of life. Depression clearly demonstrates the relationship between the body and the mind, for as the mind becomes depressed the body loses its vitality and health.

What are the common symptoms?

• Change in appetite leading to either weight gain or weight loss
• Loss of energy and feeling tired all the time
• Loss of interest in sex
• Loss of affection for your friends and family
• Loss of enjoyment and enthusiasm for life
• Loss of self-confidence
• Aches and pains for no apparent reason
• Mood swings and irritability
• Physical inactivity or hyperactivity
• Insomnia or excessive sleeping
• Feeling worthless or having inappropriate feelings of guilt
• Not being able to think or concentrate
• Thinking of death or suicide

If you have four or more of these symptoms you must contact your medical doctor. Nearly 25% of the population experiences some degree of clinical depression in their lifetime, which may require medical help.

Important to remember

If you suffer from severe depression then a course of anti-depressants can be life saving.

What are the causes?

• Genetic predisposition
• Hormonal changes during and after pregnancy

• After viral infections
• Artificial sweeteners (especially aspartame)
• Food sensitivities, especially gluten (wheat, rye, oats and barley) and dairy
• Nutritional deficiencies, such as B1, B3, B6, B12, folic acid, vitamin C and essential fatty acids, especially omega 3
• Extreme stress and anxiety
• Bereavement
• Problems with personal relationships
• Lack of sunlight
• Lack of sleep
• Chronic pain
• Drug-induced depression, especially from oral contraceptives, caffeine and smoking (carbon-monoxide and nicotine), but also from other common drugs, such as beta-blockers, high blood-pressure drugs, anti-convulsants, ulcer drugs and painkillers
• Low blood sugar levels, since a drop in blood sugar levels result in an increased release of hormones that increase the glucose levels, one of them being adrenaline. If you have a sudden drop in blood sugar you will experience tremor, sweating, anxiety, increased heart rate, hunger and possibly irritability. If you have a slow decrease the symptoms are more diffuse, such as dizziness, headache, visual disturbances, confusion and emotional instability.
• Low levels of the neuro-transmitter serotonin is linked with depression. Many of the commonly used antidepressants, such as Prozac, help to increase the effect of serotonin, which helps to lift the depression and allows the brain chemistry to return to normal. Factors that can reduce serotonin levels are alcohol consumption, smoking, blood sugar imbalances (hypoglycaemia and diabetes) and nutritional deficiencies.

What are the psychosomatic causes?

Depression may be an indication that there is a deep sadness and a longing for life to be different. There may be an unwillingness to accept life as it is, a feeling of not being in control of life's events.

Underneath sadness usually lies anger, so it may indicate unresolved emotional issues that have been bottled up and are now surfacing in an attempt from the unconscious mind to allow you to deal with it. Depression is our spirit's cry for attention, an urge for us to go within and listen to what it is we are not giving ourselves that we truly need.

How can I help with the diet?

• Increase consumption of organic products, fruits, vegetables, seeds, especially linseeds for their amino acid content, and fish.
• Make sure the brain gets a constant and steady source of blood sugar; therefore eat regularly and sensibly.
• Identify a food allergy or sensitivity, especially gluten and/or dairy (see Food Allergies).

What should I avoid?

Avoid sugar, artificial sweeteners, sweets, refined foods, coffee, chocolate, cola, tea and alcohol.

Red wine and cheese are foods that contain tyramine, which may aggravate depression. They should never be consumed if you are taking anti-depressants, since they may increase your blood pressure to a dangerous level.

Which supplements and herbs help?

Various supplements may be needed depending on the deficiencies involved. But a good rule of thumb is to take a vitamin B-complex and folic acid, vitamin C, magnesium, zinc, calcium and essential fatty acids, such as evening primrose oil, flax seed oil and fish oil. The essential fatty acids help to control and regulate the brain chemistry.

Take lactobacillus acidophilus supplements to maintain a healthy gut flora.

Flower extracts can help. For mild cases try gorse for hopelessness and despair, mustard for deep gloom for no reason, pine for guilt or willow for self-pity and resentment.

St John's wort has been shown to be as effective as antidepressants in treating mild to moderate depression and it also seems to help sleep (check with your physician if you are taking other drugs). Research has shown that this remedy alters the brain chemistry in a way that improves mood.

If over age 50 try ginkgo biloba extract, but not if you are taking any blood thinning drugs or have a blood disorder.

Oats are great for balancing the nervous system and basil is a mild antidepressant.

How else can I improve my physical health?

- Stop smoking.
- Make sure you get enough sleep.
- Increase levels of exercise. Studies have shown that exercise helps in improving depression (12,13).

How can I improve my emotional, mental and spiritual health?

Watch your thoughts. They are powerful and creative. Focus on what you want, instead of what you do not want.

Practice filling your mind with positive thoughts and affirmations daily.
Meditate daily. Allow yourself to reach your inner stillness, where you have the answer to any question you may have. Meditation combined with breathing exercises is one of the most powerful ways of restoring balance within the body-mind framework. When done in combination with positive visualisations and affirmations the unconscious mind is sent clear signals of what is required of it, and it will start to make physiological changes.

A good visualisation is to see yourself as the person you wish to be. Add all the qualities you wish to have; see yourself living the life you want. Really make it vivid. Then step out of the picture, so that you see yourself in it. Place the picture into a beautiful, pink bubble and send it off into the universe. Tell yourself, "This or something better now manifests in my life, for the highest good of all concerned."

With the aid of the coaching programme release all negative emotions, limiting beliefs, and do the forgiveness exercise in relation to all key people in your life, including your parents, siblings, partners, children and friends. Also do the exercise for solving difficult problems.

Read books that empower you, such as those by Neale Donald Walsh, Anthony Robbins, Louise Hay, Shakti Gawain, Deepak Chopra, Marianne Williamson, Diana Cooper, Christopher Hansard, Caroline Myss, John Gray, The Dalai Lama and Paramahansa Yogananda.

Which therapies help?

Counseling and psychotherapy are important when there has been any history of loss, deprivation or abuse. If you are feeling sad and it does not pass after a while, seek help.

Homeopathic treatment has several remedies which can help in mild to moderate depression.

Medical herbalism has many suitable herbs, such as St John's wort and gingko biloba.

Cranial osteopathy helps by balancing the central nervous system and improving digestion. This allows the body to express a better state of health. It may also help in postnatal depression where sometimes the strain from labour can have a profound effect on the nervous system.

Tibetan, ayurvedic and Chinese medicine help by treating the central nervous system and by balancing the energy levels of the body through the use of herbs, massage and acupuncture.

Yoga and Pilates, which co-ordinates breathing, whilst performing stabilising and mobilising exercises, are useful in bringing the body and mind back into alignment, thereby improving overall health.

Hypnotherapy, NLP and well-being coaching help because very often what you think is the reason for feeling depressed may not be the actual reason. These therapies help you by uncovering the truth, so that a real change can take place, which assists you in your dealings with the world. They enable you to find a way to take charge of your life by releasing negative thought patterns, limiting beliefs and decisions and replace them with more productive strategies.

Aromatherapy oils have many documented effects on our moods.

Healing helps by balancing the emotions and restoring energy levels.

useful affirmations

"My inner being is filled with joy."

"All is perfect just as it is."

"It is now safe for me to let go of the sadness and find what is beneath."

"Life is to be lived fully in the here and now."

"The more happiness and joy I give to myself, the more I have to give to others."

"The more happiness I give, the more I receive."

Diabetes

This is a disease that affects about 3% of the UK population, and it is becoming more common. Over one million people in the UK alone have diabetes but do not know it. Over 75% of people with diabetes have type 2 diabetes. It is characterised by an intolerance to carbohydrates and can range from mild to severe. It can be due to an insufficient production of insulin in the body or a decreased cellular sensitivity to insulin.

What different types of diabetes exist?

There are three types of diabetes, insulin dependent juvenile diabetes (IDDM-Type 1); non-insulin dependent diabetes (NIDDM-Type 2) which usually has an adult onset, and gestational diabetes. There is also a sub-clinical group that has impaired glucose intolerance, but does not yet show all the classical signs of diabetes. In this group, blood glucose levels are only slightly high… but not yet abnormal.

What are the signs and symptoms?

The signs and symptoms of Type 1 diabetes are excessive thirst, a feeling of being hungry more often, increased frequency of urination, fatigue, weight loss and irritability. There may also be vomiting and nausea.

Signs and symptoms of Type 2 diabetes are excessive thirst, pins and needles and/or numbness in feet, poor wound healing, blurred vision, a family history of diabetes and obesity.

Gestational diabetes presents with excessive thirst and increased frequency of urination. There may also be an increased feeling of hunger.

What are the complications of diabetes?

• Damage to the retina, which can cause blindness
• Damage to the nervous system, which can cause pins and needles, numbness and pain in the hands and feet
• Cardiovascular disease and kidney disease
• Poor circulation leading to gangrene in limbs, which may require amputation
• Ketoacidosis
• Coma and premature death

What are the causes?

There are many probable causes to diabetes, but the exact cause is not clear. A genetic factor is likely in both Type 1 and Type 2, especially in the latter.

Type I diabetics seem to have an auto-immune involvement; they have antibodies to their own pancreatic cells, leading to damage.

Some evidence also suggests that a viral infection may be the cause in some cases. These viruses can infect the beta cells of the islets of Langerhans in the pancreas, which can then lead to decreased function and Type 1 diabetes (14).

There may be a possible link between high exposure to prescription drugs in utero and heavy antibiotic use in young children which lead to an increased risk of developing early onset diabetes (15).

Diabetes is very rare in societies where they eat a primitive and natural diet, and seems to increase in proportion to how much refined and processed food a society is eating.

Diabetes is exceptionally common in the western world and is one of the main causes of death. The sad part is that this could often be prevented if a healthier lifestyle was adopted with better diet and more exercise.

How can a high intake of refined carbohydrates lead to diabetes?

Refined carbohydrates are converted to glucose in the body and the pancreas has to secrete insulin to remove the glucose from the blood. If this is done in excess the pancreas eventually becomes too exhausted to function properly.

How can stress affect the pancreas?

The body sees stress as an emergency (fight or flight syndrome) so therefore the body instructs the adrenal glands to secrete adrenaline that help convert stored sugar in the liver and muscles back to sugar for use in the blood stream. The body does this because it thinks it needs all this sugar for energy (to run or fight). This over-burdens the pancreas, leading to exhaustion of pancreas, adrenal glands and liver.

How can obesity affect it?

Being overweight is a major cause of diabetes, especially prolonged obesity. This seems to decrease the cellular sensitivity to insulin.

What about prenatal nutrition?

Some evidence suggests that prenatal nutrition plays a role in the development of diabetes later on. The developing fetus seems to be affected if the mother has a diet of refined carbohydrates, soft drinks and sweets leading to long periods of hyperglycaemia. It has been shown that adults born in Berlin during the war and post-war period where little refined foods were available, had far less occurrence of diabetes than adults born after this period when food was readily available (16).

What are the psychosomatic causes?

In a psychosomatic context, diabetes may be an indication of not being able to balance the sweetness in our lives; either we are drowning in too much love from others, or we are feeling a lack of love within ourselves or in our lives. We may be unable to give or receive love, leaving us feeling empty and sad.

How can I help in regards to the diet?

Eat 5–6 small, healthy meals per day. This will help to stabilise blood sugar levels.

It is extremely important to make some dietary changes, both for the diabetes and to prevent the increased risk of developing cardiovascular disease. Eat a diet rich in unrefined carbohydrates, such as brown pasta, brown rice, buckwheat, millet, oats, seeds, pulses and vegetables. Organic chicken can be consumed sparingly. Eat plenty of fresh, fatty fish, such as mackerel, salmon and herring, since these help to reduce blood platelet aggregation (a cause of blood and circulatory problems).

Soya products are recommended for their excellent protein, lecithin and choline content. Lecithin helps to emulsify fat and choline helps to prevent and treat neurological complications of diabetes. Use soya milk or goat milk as substitutes for cow's milk.

Certain foods have an insulin effect on the body, such as artichokes, brussel sprouts, green beans, garlic, cucumber, soya products, oat products, fibre, green vegetables, wheat germ and avocado. Onions and garlic help to lower blood sugar levels.

Potassium broth—made of boiled potatoes, broccoli, carrots, onions and other vegetables—is very useful to help restore lost electrolytes and minerals. Drink some daily.

What should I avoid?

• Avoid all alcohol, fruit juice, sweet fruit, dried fruit, dairy products (live yoghurt is okay), sugar, chocolate, refined and processed foods: such as white bread, white pasta, white rice, biscuits, cakes. They will overburden the system and aggravate the condition.
• Avoid all caffeine (coffee, tea, cola, chocolate) since this stimulates a stress response in the body, exhausting the adrenal glands and increasing the burden on the pancreas.
• Avoid smoked or cured meats or fish. A compound in these foods is similar in structure to another compound, which has been found to destroy beta cells in animals (17).

How else can I improve my physical health?

• Hot and cold packs (see Therapies) over the pancreas as well as mid-back to stimulate circulation and nerve flow.
• Castor oil packs (see Therapies) on the abdominal area, including the liver, pancreas, spleen, stomach and intestines since diabetes often affects all these organs as well.
• Exercise daily, such as yoga, Pilates, walking, cycling or swimming (freestyle or backstroke).

Which supplements and herbs help?

• Supplement with a good B-complex. This will help to decrease the need for insulin, aid the action of insulin as well as improve carbohydrate metabolism. B6 and B12 reduce the likelihood of developing nervous system disorders.
• Vitamin E and selenium are also needed. They may help to prevent cardiovascular disease and deterioration of the retina. Vitamin E helps minimise the damage to small blood vessels and also aids circulation.
• Vitamin C with bioflavonoids is needed to transport insulin. It helps to stabilise blood

sugar levels and is required for healthy adrenal function. Bioflavonoids increase the bioavailability of vitamin C and may also help to stop the progression of diabetic cataracts.

• Zinc is involved in insulin metabolism. Occasionally a zinc deficiency may give rise to thrush or eczema. Zinc, along with vitamin C, may help heal leg ulcers.

• Manganese is needed for glucose metabolism.

• Magnesium is important for control of blood glucose levels and if deficient will increase the risk of developing cardiovascular disease.

• Chromium, 200 micrograms per day, improves the glucose clearing activity of insulin.

• Coenzyme Q10 helps to promote insulin production.

• Garlic capsules, 2–4 per day, will help to decreasing the risk of developing cardiovascular disease.

• Fenugreek seeds have been shown to lower blood sugar (18).

• Dandelion root and burdock root contain insulin, which helps the body control blood sugar levels (19).

• Ginseng taken before a meal reduces blood sugar levels (20). Ginseng should only be taken for a four-week period, followed by a period of four weeks when ginseng is not consumed.

• Evening primrose oil may help when the nervous system has been affected. Essential fatty acids are always vital to a healthy functioning body, so supplement with omega 6 (flax seed oil, olive oil, evening primrose oil) and omega 3 (fish oil and flax seed oil) daily.

• Brewer's yeast aids the production and utilisation of insulin.

• Spirulina may help to decrease the need for insulin. Take capsules or powder 2–3 times per day.

• Half a teaspoon of cinnamon has been found to lower blood sugar levels by 20% according to recent American studies (63).

How can I improve my emotional, mental and spiritual health?

Diabetes is an illness where the whole body is crying out for some relaxation and de-stressing. So please listen to it. Practice some breathing exercises and meditate for at least 20 minutes per day.

Look at all your values for personal, family and work relationships (see coaching programme). Are they happy and fulfilling? Are they balanced and based on mutual respect and love? If they are not, then release whatever limiting beliefs and negative emotions you have formed, which are stopping you from experiencing harmony within all your relationships.

With the coaching programme release all negative emotions, limiting beliefs, pain held in the body (pancreas) and do the exercises for forgiveness in relation to all key people in your life and for solving difficult problems.

How much joy and love are you experiencing in your life? How much do you love and approve of yourself? If you find that you are experiencing low self-esteem and a lack of joy, then do something about it. Everything starts in the mind, so when you change on the inside, your outside reality will change as well.

Visualise yourself in perfect health. Then send your pancreas as much love as you possibly can. Ask it when you decided to create your diabetes and for what purpose. Ask what it needs you to do, pay attention to or learn, in order for it to get better. Then act on this guidance.

Which therapies help?

Tibetan, ayurvedic and Chinese medicine and acupuncture are highly effective treatments for helping to restore health and function of the pancreas, liver, kidneys, adrenal glands and digestive tract.

Medical herbalism and homeopathy have many useful herbs and remedies.

Osteopathic and chiropractic treatment help by improving the function of the pancreas, kidneys, liver, gastrointestinal tract and adrenal glands by stimulating proper nerves and blood flow to these organs.

Reflexology, shiatzu and acupressure help by stimulating the pancreas, liver, adrenal glands and digestive tract through pressure points.

Healing is beneficial, both by working directly on the pancreas and adrenal glands, but also by balancing your emotions.

Pilates and yoga help by improving strength, flexibility and balance within the neuro-musculo-skeletal system, which aid the healthy functioning of the pancreas and digestive tract.

useful affirmations

"My life is filled with sweetness and joy."

"Everything I need already exists within me."

"I give and receive love easily and effortlessly."

Ear Infection

This can be an acute or chronic infection that affects the middle ear. If acute, it is usually bacterial and often preceded by an upper respiratory tract infection, such as a cold. Chronic cases have a swelling of the middle ear and constant pain.

What causes it?

It is usually caused by poor functioning of the eustachian tube. Various factors can aggravate this, such as:
• An infection
• A blockage with mucous due to an allergic reaction
• Trauma, such as a difficult birth, leading to retained moulding within the temporal bone, which houses the ear. This can set up a problem with the drainage of the middle ear via the eustachian tube.

Other possible causes:
• Air travel due to the pressure changes
• Very cold weather
• High altitudes
• Constant exposure to loud noises
• Poor immune system

What are the psychosomatic causes?

It may be an indication that something we are hearing is irritating or upsetting us. When it affects a child it may be due to conflict at home, at school or with peers.

What can I do to help myself?

Improve your immune system (see **Immune System**).

What can I do to help my child?

Breast-feed your baby; he will be less susceptible to infections due to the protective antibodies from your breast milk. It has been found that breast-fed infants have a much larger thymus gland (vital organ for immune system) than bottle-fed infants (40).

It is advisable to breast-feed exclusively for the first six months of a baby's life. The digestive tract is poorly developed until six months of age and it is more common to develop food allergies and sensitivities when certain foods are introduced too early, especially dairy products, wheat, egg, nuts and fowl. The breast-feeding mother may need to exclude common allergenic foods from her diet, since it can be passed on to the baby through the breast milk.

What should I avoid?

• Avoid any known food allergens, such as milk and other dairy products, nuts, wheat, corn, egg and oranges (see Food Allergies). An allergic reaction can cause a blockage of the eustachian tubes setting up a perfect environment for chronic ear infections. Many children with chronic ear infections have an allergy to food, inhalants or both.
• Avoid colourings and food additives.
• Public swimming pools
• Getting a chill
• Smoky environments, house dust, animal hair and fungus spores can irritate the condition. Remove all wall-to-wall carpets, do not smoke in the house, clean regularly using natural cleaning products, and remove all signs of damp.

What should I do in regards to antibiotics?

Often antibiotics are prescribed for acute ear infections, because of the risk of the infection spreading to the brain and mastoid. It is always important to be examined by a medical doctor to establish how serious the infection is; however, children receiving antibiotics seem to have more recurrent infections than those who do not. Antibiotics also increase the risk of fungal and yeast infections. If antibiotics have to be given, also give probiotic supplements, such as lactobacillus acidophilus, to help normalise gut functioning, since antibiotics wipe out the friendly and necessary gut flora. This supplement needs to be taken at least three hours apart from the antibiotics. It is sometimes best to wait until after the course of antibiotics has finished to take the probiotics.

How can I help prevent ear infections?

• Take echinacea, zinc, vitamin C with bioflavonoids, beta-carotene, propolis and garlic. The cochlear needs vitamin A to function properly, and vitamin E can help improve hearing.
• Take a multivitamin and mineral supplement daily (tablet or liquid).
• Take essential fatty acids daily, such as fish oil or flaxseed oil.
• If given antibiotics also take lactobacillus acidophilus capsules/powder.
• Humidifiers seem to help, probably because low humidity may contribute to an ear infection, since it may decrease the ventilation or dry the lining of the eustachian tube. This could increase the secretions and reduce the ability to clear the fluid from the ear.

What can I do when an infection is present?

Soak diluted mullein oil on a piece of cotton wool and put this in the affected ear. Alternatively, use diluted lavender oil.

Soak some cotton wool in a little garlic oil diluted with grape seed oil (or other carrier oil) and place in the ear to help draw out an infection. (Be careful not to let the garlic oil touch any skin surface).

An onion poultice applied locally can help.

Bach Rescue Remedy cream can be applied around the ears to decrease the inflammation and soothe emotions.

It is sometimes helpful to wrap a few ice cubes in a cloth and apply it to the affected ear. This helps to decrease the inflammation and aid in decongestion. Sometimes heat may seem to relieve the pain, but it often increases the inflammatory response, which is not desirable.

Stimulate the thymus gland by doing hot and cold treatment over the lower part of the throat. Soak a cloth in hot/warm water. Place it on the throat and upper chest for 30–60 seconds, remove it and place a cold cloth on the throat and upper chest for 10–20 seconds. Repeat 2–3 times a few times per day. This is a highly effective treatment for improving the immune system.

Make sure you and your child are well dressed to avoid chills. In winter, make sure to wear a hat that covers the ears.

If your child has an ear infection, it is useful to have him sleep with the head slightly elevated so that the eustachian tubes can drain naturally.

How can I improve my or my child's emotional, mental and spiritual health?

When it comes to the emotional, mental and spiritual health of a child, it is obviously important to look at the family dynamics. Children pick up any negative emotions, such as anger, sadness, fear, guilt and hurt from their environment, even if the parents are trying to cover it up to protect the child. When we are very young we react instinctively to our environment and take things very personally. That is why children always believe it is their fault if the parents are arguing or upset. The most appropriate action here is for the parents to release any emotional issues within themselves that may be upsetting the child.

If you are suffering from ear infections, use the coaching programme to release all your negative emotions, limiting beliefs and emotional pain held in the body or caused by unwanted states and behaviours and do the forgiveness exercise.

If something is irritating you in your environment, try to see the situation from the other person's perspective and do the exercise for solving difficult problems.

Which therapies help?

Cranial osteopathy helps by reducing any retained moulding and compression within the temporal bone, assisting with the drainage of the mucous build up, as well as improving the functioning of the eustachian tubes. Normally the response to treatment is a gradual improvement. It is a good sign when a cold does not develop into an ear infection, when it normally would have.

Homeopathy – homeopathic eardrops can be very useful, such as pulsatilla and belladonna. Homeopathic remedies work on an energetic level, so they can be of great help to address any emotional imbalances within the body-mind framework. See a qualified homeopath for appropriate advice.

Medical herbalism – there are several herbs, such as echinacea, goldenseal and liquorice that can assist in improving the immune system, which will help the body resist infection. Consult a qualified herbalist for appropriate advice.

Aromatherapy – various oils have a calming effect on our emotions, such as Roman chamomile and lavender. It may help to put a few drops on a piece of cotton wool underneath the child's pillow at night.

Healing may be of great benefit, especially if the whole family receives it.

Kinesiology helps by establishing if any food sensitivities are present and also aids in balancing the musculo-skeletal system.

Tibetan, ayurvedic and Chinese medicine help to improve the immune system and aid the drainage of the ears.

Reflexology, shiatzu and acupressure help by stimulating pressure points relating to the ears, digestive tract and nervous system.

NLP, hypnotherapy and well-being coaching help by releasing repressed negative emotions and limiting beliefs. If a young child is suffering with recurrent ear infections, it may be appropriate for the parents to look at themselves to see if something they are doing is causing the child to feel stressed, in which case these therapies can help.

Useful affirmations

"It is safe for me to hear everything that goes on in my life."

"I am filled with love and light. All is well in my world."

Eczema

This is a chronic inflammatory condition of the skin affecting 2–8% of adults (higher percentage in children). The skin itches and is dry and thickened. Various lesions can occur, such as papules, redness, scaling with tiny blisters and weeping of fluid. There is often a family history of asthma, hay fever or eczema.

What commonly causes it?

There seems to be evidence to suggest that eczema is a reaction to a food allergen. Many people improve when they adopt an elimination diet, excluding all common food allergens, such as dairy, fish, soya, egg, corn, peanut, wheat and citrus. In children there is a strong link with dairy intolerance. This can be triggered by lack of breast-feeding, using infant formula based on cow milk, early or improper weaning, or if the mother is eating the allergenic food during pregnancy or whilst breast feeding.

What seems to aggravate it?

Stress, low stomach acid and a decreased immunological ability to kill bacteria lead to an increased risk of developing other skin infections.

What are the psychosomatic causes?

In a psychosomatic context eczema may be a representation of dysfunctional mental and emotional patterns that want to be released through the skin so that a new person can emerge. It may be an indication that we are frustrated with ourselves and the world, so much so that the skin—the part of our being that is the first contact with the world around us—becomes inflamed. Eczema may also indicate bottled-up feelings that need to be let out; when feelings are not allowed to be heard and understood, they can come out through the skin. It is often aggravated by hidden emotions, especially in individuals who are unable to communicate their feelings and be understood, such as children.

How can I help my child in regards to diet?

Breast-feed for at least six months, especially if there is a family history of eczema, asthma or hay fever.

Wean the child slowly and introduce one food group at a time. Wait a few days for any signs of reaction before introducing another food group. Do not introduce cow milk and eggs for the first three years of the child's life if there is a family history of asthma, eczema, hay fever or an allergy to these food substances. Never introduce peanuts until the child is three years old.

In children, milk and other dairy products are usually the main allergen. If you are not breast-feeding, try switching to a soya based milk, or a goat milk formula. Another common allergen is wheat. Avoid all artificial colourings, flavourings or preservatives. Sometimes fermented foods, such as vinegar, soya sauce and alcohol (as in tinctures) may be the offending allergen.

How can I help myself in regards to the diet?

It is important to eliminate all common food allergens and then adopt a rotation diet until the condition has cleared up. Slowly the allergenic foods can once again be introduced into the diet (see **Allergies**).

What else can I do (both adults and children)?

Bach Rescue Remedy cream is good for dry skin, whilst urtica urens ointment may help to relieve itching. Evening primrose oil has been shown to reduce itching and speed up the healing process. Aloe vera gel helps to heal the skin, as do creams with chamomile, liquorice or witch hazel.

Apply olive oil after a bath, whilst the skin is still warm. A few drops of lavender oil in the bath can help to soothe the skin.

Make sure the bedroom is of a natural flooring, such as wood. Carpets attracts dust mite, which has been shown to aggravate eczema.

If the condition seems to improve in nature and gets worse in a city, then environmental pollutants may be at cause.

Which supplements help?

To reduce inflammation, take flax seed oil (from the age of six months), as well as vitamin C and bioflavonoids. Vitamin A helps the repair and development of the skin, and zinc is needed for essential fatty acid metabolism, which is important to decrease the inflammatory response. B-complex is important for the healthy functioning of the skin. Vitamin E may also be needed.

Take a good quality multivitamin and mineral formula, an anti-oxidant, a B-complex and flaxseed oil daily.

Lactobacillus acidophilus capsules or powder help the proper functioning of the intestines.

What about any side effects to common orthodox treatments?

Many steroid preparations used to treat eczema have severe side effects, such as thinning of the skin and osteoporosis (thinning of bones). Many use antibiotics to decrease the risk of infections of the skin, which sets up a fertile ground for candida infections (makes eczema worse). Patients using systemic steroids, who have not had measles or chickenpox, can be in danger of dying from eczema because steroids severely affect the immune system. About 30 patients die in the UK from this complication each year (21).

How can I improve my or my child's emotional, mental or spiritual health?

Stress reduction is very important. If your child suffers from eczema, then make sure the home environment is as calm and peaceful as possible. Limit unnecessary excitement to an absolute minimum, and stick to a daily routine. Make sure your child gets plenty of sleep and has lots of fun, so that he is able to feel happy and calm.

Adults should practice daily meditation and breathing exercises. This balances the nervous system, which aids digestion. A useful visualisation is to send your skin as much love as you possibly can—as a healing balm—making it healthy, smooth and glowing.

With the aid of the coaching programme release all negative emotions and limiting beliefs.

Which therapies help?

Medical herbalism has many useful herbs, such as stinging nettle, chickweed and burdock.

Homeopathic remedies help, such as calendula and sulphur.

Tibetan, ayurvedic and Chinese medicine and acupuncture help by improving the immune system and digestion.

Healing is highly beneficial, since eczema is closely linked to our emotional well-being.

NLP, hypnotherapy and well-being coaching help to release repressed negative emotions.

Useful affirmations

"Peace and joy fill my body and mind."

"It is now safe for me to let my feelings out."

"I am loveable and wonderful just as I am."

"It is safe for me to be myself."

Food Allergies and Sensitivities

A food allergy will mount a classic antigen-antibody response to the particular food that is causing the allergy. It can lead to anaphylactic shock and be potentially life threatening. A food sensitivity is a reaction to a particular food, but without the antigen-antibody response.

What are common symptoms of an immediate response?

Swelling, watery eyes, wheezing, hives and skin rashes

What are symptoms of a delayed response?

Some symptoms take time to develop, usually 36–72 hours after the allergenic food has been eaten. It can affect any of the body's systems, giving rise to a wide range of problems, such as skin rashes, eczema, psoriasis, acne, dark circles under eyes, sinusitis, chronic infections, diarrhoea, constipation, stomach ulcers, constant tiredness, headaches, arthritis, menstrual disorders, anxiety, depression, mental confusion and insomnia. In children it can be the underlying cause of problems with colic, bladder control, diarrhoea, constipation, hyperactivity, eczema and recurrent ear and chest infections.

What is the difference between cyclical and fixed food allergies?

A cyclical allergy develops slowly and is often due to repetitive eating of the same food, making the body sensitive to it. By avoiding the allergenic food for a long period (4–6 months) sensitivity often disappears and the food can then be tolerated again if eaten in moderation. A fixed food allergy is life long, and never improves with time.

Why are allergies and sensitivities on the increase in children?

It may be due to a variety of factors leading to increased stress on the immune system, such as:
• Genetic. It has been shown that children of parents who have a food allergy/sensitivity have an increased risk of developing an allergy/sensitivity themselves (if both parents are allergic, the child has a 67% risk of developing the same allergy).
• Eating nut products or other allergenic foods while pregnant or breastfeeding, since this may cause an allergy in the baby.
• Premature birth, since the digestive tract is not fully formed

• Not breastfeeding. Many infants cannot tolerate baby formulas, especially the ones derived from cow milk, since those proteins are hard to digest. Breast milk contains important protective factors, which decrease the risk of developing an allergy.

• Improper and premature weaning. No child should be weaned before six months of age, since the digestive tract does not mature until that time. Certainly gluten, wheat, corn and dairy products should not be used as the first weaning foods. Cow milk should not be given at all until the child is at least 12 months, or three years if there is a history of asthma, eczema or hay fever in the family. Nut products should not be given to any child under the age of three years.

• Repetitive use of antibiotics, since this wipes out the healthy gut flora

• Food additives and colourings increase the risk of developing an allergy/sensitivity, and they affect the central nervous system—especially in children—making them prone to hyperactivity, poor concentration and mood disturbances.

• Vaccination toxicity, since this may be linked with poor gut function, setting up the grounds for allergies/sensitivities to develop. MMR vaccine seems to be the one causing most of the debate.

What are the possible causes for the increase in adults?

• Genetic manipulation of foods, chemicals and pesticides, various industrial chemicals, metals and pollutants all affect our immune system making us more prone to develop allergies/ sensitivities.

• Candida, parasite or fungi overgrowth impair the functioning of the digestive tract.

• Digestive problems and liver dysfunction.

• Excessive alcohol intake can lead to liver dysfunction, nutritional deficiencies and digestive problems.

• Improper diet, such as eating the same foods all the time or having a very acid forming diet

• Large consumption of caffeine and tea stimulate the adrenal glands to produce stress hormones, leading to lowered immune function.

• Any illness leading to a severe disruption of the immune system

• Stress—physical, emotional and mental—impairs the immune system.

What are the psychosomatic causes?

In a psychosomatic context allergies may represent our inability to digest our environment, our reality. It is something we are not tolerating, something that is causing us irritation and that we have an emotional response to (watery eyes, stuffy nose, skin rashes). Who or what are we reacting against? It may indicate deep-seated fear and suppressed emotions that need to have an outlet.

How can you diagnose an allergy?

One way is through elimination diets. This involves the patient eating only non-allergenic foods for 1–4 weeks until all symptoms have disappeared. Then one food is reintroduced to see if a reaction occurs (can take 1–3 days), then the next food is reintroduced four days later, and so on. This is a very reliable method, but demands determination from the patient.

Another way is the blood test, which is often used by complementary practitioners. It is very reliable, since it can measure IgE, IgG, IgG4 and IgA antibodies, and therefore it can identify many different types of allergies.

Skin-prick tests are commonly used in orthodox medicine. It only measures IgE antibodies and therefore can only pick up about 10–15% of all allergies.

The reintroduction of food substances should never be used in patients with severe allergic reactions, since this could lead to a potentially life-threatening situation.

How can I help myself?

Fasts can be used as a sure way of eliminating all allergy producing foods and then reintroducing them one at a time. Fasting should only be done under supervision and is not suitable for everyone.

Elimination diets where the allergic foods are avoided for at least 4–5 days, then are reintroduced one at a time to see if they produce any reactions, can be very useful. This can be quite difficult to do, since many common food allergens are used in preparation of food, such as wheat, corn, soy and egg. So always read the labels and avoid eating out during this phase. Only undertake to do this under the supervision of a qualified practitioner.
Rotation diets are useful once the allergy producing foods have been eliminated. Eating the same type of food only every four days is a good way of making sure that your diet is varied.

Make sure that the food you eat is organic.

Drink plenty of pure water to help the body flush out toxins and waste products.

What should I avoid?

• Avoid smoking, drinking coffee, tea, chocolate and alcohol since these produce a stress response
• Eliminate all sugar and yeast products if there is any suspicion of candida albicans
• Avoid contact with household pets
• Remove all wall-to-wall carpets, since they attract dust mite and dirt. Instead use wooden, ceramic or laminated flooring, which is easier to clean (with natural cleaning products).

Which supplements and herbs help?

Stimulate the immune system (see **Immune System**). Take a good multivitamin and mineral.

Lactobacillus acidophilus (non-dairy) capsules may be useful to restore gut flora.

Take essential fatty acids such as flax seed oil (omega 3 and 6) or evening primrose oil (omega 6) and fish oil (omega 3) daily.

Garlic capsules (2–6) daily.

How can I improve my emotional, mental and spiritual health?

• Decrease the normal stress response in your body by practising daily meditation, breathing exercises and other forms of relaxation.
• Have fun. Practice the art of laughing at yourself and at life.
• Follow your dreams. Listen to your inner guidance and act on it. Life wants you to be happy, balanced, full of enthusiasm, and true to your inner self.
• If someone or something is annoying you, look at it closely. What is it mirroring back to you? Is it highlighting an aspect of yourself you don't like, or is it perhaps giving you an opportunity to deal with it appropriately this time? Once you have found the understanding, the irritation you felt in regards to the person or situation will disappear. With the coaching programme do the exercises for solving difficult problems and for releasing negative emotions.

Which therapies help?

Tibetan, ayurvedic and Chinese medicine help by improving the immune system and digestive tract.

Homeopathy and herbal medicine have several remedies and herbs which are helpful.

Osteopathy and chiropractic help by balancing the neuro-musculo-skeletal structure, which aids the function of the immune system and the digestive tract.

Healing helps to balance the emotions and to restore energy levels.

NLP, hypnotherapy and well-being coaching help by improving emotional and mental balance, thereby reducing excess stress within the body.

Useful affirmations

"The world is a fun and safe place to live in."

"I am filled with light and love."

"It is now safe and easy for me to establish my boundaries with love."

Gout

This is a recurrent form of arthritis caused by an increased concentration of uric acid, which accumulates in the joints, tendons, intestines, kidneys and other body tissues, causing intense pain.

What are the causes?

The causes of gout can be primary or secondary. Primary gout accounts for about 90% of cases and often the exact cause is not known. In secondary gout the increased uric acid levels may be due to a primary disease process or as a side-effect of various drugs, such as chemotherapy, certain diuretics and even low doses of aspirin.

The most common causes are:
• High consumption of meat, sugar, refined carbohydrates, coffee and alcohol
• Low intake of fresh fruit and vegetables
• Obesity
• Decreased kidney clearance of uric acid. This can be due to a variety of causes, such as intrinsic kidney disease, alcoholism, diabetic ketoacidosis, lead poisoning, certain medications (thiazides diuretics, salicylates, penicillin, insulin etc.) and various other renal problems.
• Increased production of purines, which can be due to poor dietary intake (see above), cancer, chronic anaemia, certain drugs, psoriasis, stress leading to adrenal exhaustion and enzyme deficiency.

Some diseases may also increase the risk of developing gout, such as thyroid or parathyroid problems, cardiovascular disease and hypertension.

What are the signs and symptoms?

It typically affects one joint, commonly the joint of the big toe and the first attack usually occurs at night. Other symptoms are headaches, fever, chills, constipation, indigestion, kidney stones formed by uric acid, heart problems and genetic predisposition. Soft tissue nodules that are chalk-like in appearance may form in the earlobes, tendons and cartilage. Over 90-95 percent of sufferers are men over the age of thirty.

Why has it been called the rich man's disease?

It has been called this, since many attacks follow an indulgence of consuming huge quantities of meat and wine. This is because meat contains high levels of purines, which increase the uric acid concentration of the blood, and alcohol gives a decreased renal (kidney) clearance of uric acid and an increased uric acid production.

What are the psychosomatic causes?

In a psychosomatic context, increased uric acid production may be seen as increased activity of negative thought patterns and behaviours. As these build up they start to impair the functioning of the affected peripheral joint (peripheral joints represent our ability to move with ease through life). Gout may therefore represent a person that is negative, angry and constantly looking for faults in others and in himself.

How can I help in regards to the diet?

Increase consumption of low-purine foods, such as green vegetables, fruit, rice, millet, cornbread, eggs, goat's milk and goat's yoghurt.
Eat plenty of white deep-sea fish.
Eat plenty of red and blue berries, such as cherries, blueberries, strawberries and hawthorn berries, since these have shown to be very effective in reducing the uric acid levels and in preventing further attacks. This is due to their anthocyanidins and proanthocyanidins content, which are very effective in preventing collagen destruction.
Drink plenty of filtered water (at least 6-8 glasses) to help flush out toxins and increase uric acid excretion. This will help to prevent the build up of uric acid crystals.

What should I avoid?

• Avoid all alcohol
• Avoid cow milk products.
• Decrease intake of foods that increase uric acid production, such as saturated fats, meat, herring, mackerel, anchovies, sardines, mushrooms, yeast, oat porridge, spices, asparagus, shellfish and sweetbreads.

How else can I improve my physical health?

• A detox program may be required. Always consult your medical doctor and naturopath before doing this.
• If you are overweight you may need to loose weight, since uric acid levels have shown to decrease significantly as the weight drops.
• Hot epsom salt baths to aid in detoxification. Never do during an acute episode.
• Hot and cold showers to stimulate circulation. Castor oil packs to the liver to aid detoxification (see therapies).

Which herbs and supplements help?

• Supplement with vitamin C (small dose only of 500 mg as large doses can lead to increased uric acid production).
• Vitamin E inhibits production of leukotrienes that are involved in the inflammatory response.
• Selenium helps to potentiate the effect of vitamin E.
• Bioflavonoid, especially quercetin, helps to inhibit uric acid production.
• Folic acid, which inhibits the enzyme that is involved in production of uric acid.
• Cod liver oil capsules, since omega 3 fatty acids have shown to decrease the inflammatory response. Do not use fish oil made from salmon, since they are high in purines. Flax seed oil will also be useful.
• Devil's claw may be of use in reducing uric acid levels, decreasing joint pain as well as having an anti-inflammatory action. It should only be used as a short term solution.

How can I improve my emotional, mental and spiritual health?

• Train yourself to always look for the positive in others and in any situation in life.
• Release old, negative emotions with the aid of

the coaching programme. Let go of all past perceived wrong doings. If someone did something bad 10 years ago, realise this was 10 years ago, and that it has nothing to do with you now. • Release it and let it go. By doing this you allow yourself to live in the now and not in the past.

• Practice breathing exercises and meditation daily. This allows you to regularly let go of negativity, while connecting with the infinite love within.

• A useful meditation is to go within to that still inner place. Place your awareness in your heart and connect with the deep love that lives there.

• Feel this love and then let this love flow with your blood to every cell of your body. Keep doing this until you feel thoroughly peaceful. Then send love out from your heart to your family, friends and everyone you know. Keep doing this until you feel complete.

• Do the Forgiveness exercise for everyone you feel any negative emotions towards.

Which therapies help?

Tibetan, ayurvedic and Chinese medicine and acupuncture can help greatly with aiding the body to clear the excess uric acid, as well as helping it to improve its overall health.

Homeopathy - there are several remedies, which can be of benefit, such as belladonna (when there is a sudden onset, with swelling, inflammation and pain), arnica montana (when the pain has a bruised feeling) and ledum palustre (when foot and big toe are very swollen). There are many more suitable remedies, so please see a practitioner.

Healing can help by allowing the individual to let go of stored negative emotions, and balance both the emotions and the nervous system.

Medical herbalism has many useful herbs. See a practitioner for specific advice.

Osteopathic and chiropractic treatment help

by improving the function of the elimination organs, such as the liver and kidneys so as to help the body in decreasing its uric acid content, as well as treating any other structural and functional problems which might aggravate the arthritic condition.

Reflexology, shiatzu and acupressure help by aiding the kidney and liver in their function. NLP, hypnotherapy and well-being coaching help in pain control, as an efficient way of releasing unwanted states and behaviours and letting go of past negative emotions.

useful affirmations

"I let go of the old and embrace the new."

"I now find peace within myself and the way I relate to others."

"Love and peace fills my heart and blood."

Haemorrhoids

Haemorrhoids are enlarged, distended veins of the haemorrhoidal plexus around the anus. They can be internal, external or mixed (when an internal haemorrhoid has prolapsed and descends below the anal sphincter).

What are the symptoms?

Haemorrhoids usually give bright, red blood on the toilet tissue with the passing of stools. They may also cause inflammation around the anus, which leads to itching and discomfort. Only a haemorrhoid that is ulcerated, prolapsed or thrombosed will give rise to pain (at times severe).

When do they usually occur?

They are extremely common in the western

world, especially after the age of fifty, due to a high incidence of constipation. Most people start to show symptoms in their thirties, but often the haemorrhoids have already developed in their twenties, or even in childhood. Haemorrhoids are rare in countries where an unrefined, high fibre diet is consumed (22).

What are the causes?

Increased intra-abdominal pressure, from straining on the toilet, lifting heavy objects, coughing, sneezing, vomiting (such as in bulimia nervosa), during pregnancy, and portal hypertension (cirrhosis of liver).

Veins in the rectal area have no valves, so if there is congestion of blood flow, such as can occur during prolonged sitting, haemorrhoids can be formed.

What are the psychosomatic causes?

Haemorrhoids may be an indication of an individual who is holding on to past emotional issues, such as anger, guilt or sadness, while at the same time trying to force them out by straining and pushing. Therefore an inner conflict arises of wanting to hold on, while at the same time pushing away. There may be a fear of letting go; a fear of new demands being placed upon us as we release the past. This might sometimes be seen in abusive relationships, where the abused feels a deep anger and resentment towards the perpetrator, but at the same time is holding on to the relationship out of fear of being alone, or out of a need of still wanting to be loved and accepted (common feeling in children who are being abused by their parents).

How can I help in regards to the diet?

Address the problem of constipation. Haemorrhoids are rare in countries where the food is unrefined with high fibre content (see **Constipation**).

Proanthocyanidin and anthocyanidin-rich foods are beneficial to strengthen the tissues of the veins. Eat lots of blue and red berries, such as strawberries, blueberries and cherries. Also eat plenty of flavonoid-rich foods, such as berries and citrus fruit, since these also help to increase the strength of the veins.

Pumpkin seeds (zinc and essential fatty acids) and sunflower seeds (essential fatty acids) help tissues heal and reduce inflammation.

A tablespoon of linseeds and olive oil daily aid gut motility and softens the stools.

Which supplements and herbs help?

Psyllium husk capsules or guar gum may be needed to increase fibre content. Studies have shown that increased fibre intake can reduce symptoms of haemorrhoids (23).
Vitamin C, bioflavonoids, vitamin A and E, B-complex and zinc aid tissue repair.

How else can I improve my physical health?

• Do not strain when sitting on the toilet, since this increases the intra-abdominal pressure.
• Avoid standing or sitting for prolonged periods, and avoid heavy lifting.
• Hot and cold sitz baths improve circulation and aid recovery of affected tissues.
• Locally applied cold packs are good during acute phases, especially when there is inflammation.
• Witch hazel cream applied locally is good for all cases. Also useful is a lemon juice compress.
• Yoga and Pilates exercises focusing mostly on strengthening the pelvic floor, aiding the function of the diaphragm, improving spinal mobility for the segments responsible for healthy nerve flow to the digestive tract (top of neck,

mid back and sacrum) and re-aligning the balance between the pelvis and lower back.

How can I improve my emotional, mental and spiritual health?

Use the coaching programme to release all negative emotions, limiting beliefs, emotional pain held in the body or caused by unwanted states and behaviours, and do the forgiveness exercise in relation to all the key people in your life, and if needed for a specific traumatic event. This frees you from the past, and enables you to fully live in the now as a happy and free individual.

Practice saying 'no' with love. Learn to prioritise your own needs and set boundaries.

Find out your inner wishes and needs. What is important to you in life? What qualities and experiences do you need to be happy and fulfilled? Write them down, and then look for ways to make this your reality.

Daily meditation strengthens your connection with your inner wisdom and calms your mind.

Which therapies help?

Pilates helps by improving the neuro-musculo-skeletal balance, which aids circulation and venous drainage as well as improving the function of the diaphragm.

Tibetan, Chinese and ayurvedic medicine help improve circulation and bowel function.

Reflexology, shiatzu and acupressure help improve function of the digestive tract, diaphragm and circulation.

Osteopathy and chiropractic help improve the neuro-musculo-skeletal balance, digestion and the function of the diaphragm.

Homeopathic remedies, such as calcarea fluorica (for bleeding and itching from the haemorrhoids) and aloe socotrina (when haemorrhoids

are swollen and protruding).

Healing helps to balance the emotions.

NLP, hypnotherapy and well-being coaching help to release negative emotions and limiting beliefs, change unwanted states and behaviours and set up positive goals for the future.

Useful affirmations

"It is now safe for me to release the past and embrace the now with joy and love."

"As I release the past I make room for my future to be filled with happiness."

"As I forgive the past I set myself free."

"I now choose to do that which fills me with joy. I am worth it."

Warning: Always contact a medical doctor if you have any rectal bleeding, to rule out any sinister causes.

Hay Fever

This is a seasonal allergic rhinitis, which is an allergic reaction to inhaled allergens, such as pollen from grass and trees, or fungus spores. Some individuals suffer from non-seasonal allergens, such as dust, which can cause year-round rhinitis.

What are the signs and symptoms?

Watery, itchy eyes, runny nose with sneezing, sore throat, tightness in the chest and tiredness. It is commonly associated with asthma, and often exists in families who have one or more of the atopic conditions: asthma, eczema or hay fever.

What are the causes?

It is usually caused by a weakened immune system, which can be due to a variety of factors, such as food allergies/sensitivities, additives and colourings in food, stress, digestive disorders, smoking, poor drinking habits (too much caffeine and/or alcohol).

What are the psychosomatic causes?

Hay fever may indicate blocked emotions or that there is something in our environment we are having an emotional reaction against (watery, itchy eyes, sore throat and tightness in the chest).

How can I help in regards to the diet?

For a young child:
• In families where one or more of the atopic conditions exist it is important to wean the child properly and not too early (see Food Allergies).
• Breastfeed until the child is 6 months and during that time the mother should eat a healthy diet, avoiding all the common food allergens, colourings and pesticides.
• Avoid giving cow milk until the child is at least three years of age. This is because dairy is mucous forming, which may aggravate all three conditions.

For an older child and adults:
• Eat organic as much as possible.
• Increase consumption of fresh fruits (except citrus), vegetables, seeds, millet and pulses.
• Drink plenty of filtered water daily.

What should I avoid?

• Eliminate all food allergens, especially dairy, chocolate, wheat, citrus, nuts, eggs and shellfish.
• Avoid all colourings and preservatives.
• Avoid pesticides as much as possible.
• Avoid white sugar and salt. (Instead use brown sugar, honey and herbal salt, but sparingly).
• Avoid caffeine, tea and alcohol.

Which supplements and herbs may help?

• Vitamin C with bioflavonoids, A, E, B-complex, zinc, selenium, echinacea, goldenseal and garlic all help to improve immune function (see **Immune System**).
• Essential fatty acids, such as flax seed oil or evening primrose oil help by improving the function of the nervous system thereby helping the overall health of the body.

How else can I improve my physical health?

It may be necessary to go on a detox fast. Only undertake to do this under the supervision of a naturopath or nutritional therapist.

Hot and cold packs (see **Therapies**) to the thymus stimulate the immune system.
Epsom salt baths aid in eliminating toxins.

Castor oil packs, especially to the liver, are useful as they help to detoxify the body.

How can I improve my emotional, mental and spiritual health?

Daily meditation and relaxation will help you to balance your mind and emotions, as well as improve your immune system.

Are you holding on to negative emotions or limiting beliefs? If so, take the time now to release them with the help of the coaching programme.

Is there anything or anyone in your life you are reacting against? Look at this situation, and see how much negative energy is being poured into it. Are you now willing to let it go? Are you ready to forgive, so that you free yourself from the emotional charge of this drama? With the help of the coaching programme do the exercises for forgiveness (in relation to everyone involved in this situation) and for solving difficult problems.

Meditate on your hay fever. Ask it what its highest purpose is for you, and what it wants you to pay attention to, know or learn for it to improve. Then act on this guidance.

Which therapies help?

Tibetan, ayurvedic and Chinese medicine are very efficient treatments for restoring the balance of the immune system and digestive tract through the use of herbs, massage and acupuncture.

Osteopathy and chiropractic help by improving the function of the digestive tract, liver and immune system.

Cranial osteopathy helps by balancing the digestive, nervous and immune systems.

Reflexology, acupressure and shiatzu help improve the immune system and digestive tract by stimulating pressure points.

Healing is useful for restoring energy and for balancing the emotions.

Medical herbalism helps through a variety of herbs, which aim to improve the function of the immune system and balance the nervous system.

Homeopathic remedies, such as allium cepa (watery eyes, tickling cough and nasal discharge), nux vomica (a stuffed or runny nose and a tickling cough) and wyethia (itching in the mouth, behind nose or in throat). Many more remedies may be suitable.

Kinesiology helps by establishing any allergies and musculo-skeletal imbalances that are affecting the health of the body.

NLP, hypnotherapy and well-being coaching help by releasing negative emotions, limiting beliefs and changing unwanted states and behaviours. This frees your body and mind from inner tension, which makes more energy available for the overall function of the body, including the immune system.

Useful affirmations

"As I forgive others I set myself free."

"As I release negative emotions from the past I am able to connect with my inner happiness."

"I now release the past and embrace my new life."

Headaches

About 98% of the western adult population suffer from a non-serious headache on a regular basis. 2–5% of adults can have pain lasting for more than 15 days per month. The most common is a tension headache, which is usually felt behind the eyes or at the back of the head. Other types of headaches are migraines and cluster headaches.

What causes a tension headache?

It is normally caused by contraction of the head and neck muscles and/or joint restrictions in the upper part of the neck. It is a common response to stress, anxiety, anger, poor posture and lack of sleep.

What is a migraine?

Migraines can be classic or common. A classic migraine will give a severe throbbing pain, usually on one side of the head, often accompanied by nausea and sometimes vomiting. Before the headache comes on the patient experiences pro-dromal symptoms, such as blurred vision, light sensitivity, dizziness and numbness to one side of the body. With a common migraine there is pain usually on one side of the head, but without any warning signs. This type of headache can last between 1–3 days.

What causes a migraine?

A typical migraine is caused by an initial vaso-constriction (blood vessels constrict) limiting the blood flow to the brain, followed by vasodi-lation, which increases the blood flow leading to a throbbing headache. A tension headache is caused by a vasoconstriction only.

Food intolerance is probably the most likely cause of migraine. Common foods that can induce a migraine attack are chocolate, cheese, alcohol (especially red wine), cow milk, shell-fish, citrus fruit, coffee and tea. Of these, choco-late, cheese and alcohol most commonly seem to precipitate migraine attacks.

What are cluster headaches?

Cluster headaches are very painful and are usu-ally localised around one eye. They mainly affect men who are heavy smokers and lead very stressful lives. The headaches tend to occur in clusters lasting 1–3 days and recur every few months.

What are other common causes of headaches?

• Stress and anxiety
• Muscle spasm and neck joint restrictions (especially with tension headaches)
• In children who experience headaches around the age of 7–8 years it is often due to retained moulding within the skull from birth trauma or a bad fall
• Food allergies
• Difficulty expressing emotions (usually anger)

• Sensitivity to blood sugar levels (reactive hypoglycaemia). This is especially common in headaches felt in the morning, where blood sugar levels drop at night
• Dental disorders, including grinding teeth at night
• Refractive errors in the eyes requiring glasses
• TMJ dysfunction (jaw)
• Poor diet and nutritional deficiencies
• Excessive intake of salt, MSG or aspartame
• Alcohol or drug abuse
• Withdrawal symptoms from caffeine
• Smoking, since nicotine causes blood vessels to constrict, while carbon monoxide causes them to dilate. This can create cluster headaches and migraines.

What are other less common causes?

Hormonal imbalance, hypertension, sinusitis, anaemia, meningeal irritation, head trauma causing traction or displacement of dura, blood vessels and nerves, dilation of intra- and extra-cranial vessels (common in migraines), increased intra-cranial pressure, glaucoma, toxic colon and/or liver, post traumatic pain, post-herpetic neuralgia (nerve pain after shingles), atypical facial pain, brain tumour and temporal arteritis.

What are the psychosomatic causes?

In a psychosomatic context a headache may be an indication of bottled up emotions that are not being let out or thoughts that may need to be voiced but are repressed. Instead we grind our teeth, lock our jaws, tighten our neck mus-cles and soldier on, creating insurmountable pressure within us. It may also indicate a ten-dency of putting ourself down and constantly criticising ourself and others. Migraines are often seen in people who are perfectionists, who rarely feel that they are perfect just as they are.

How can I help in regards to diet?

Eat organic as much as possible to decrease amount of toxins being ingested.

Increase food consumption of vegetable oils, fish oils, blackcurrant seed oil, garlic and onion, which decrease platelet aggregation and provide anti-inflammatory substances to prevent vaso-constriction.

What should I avoid?

• Avoid any known food allergens (see Food Allergies), colourings and artificial sweeteners
• Especially avoid alcohol, chocolate, cheese, shellfish and citrus fruits
• Avoid stress and harbouring negative feelings
• Resolve emotional issues as soon as possible

Which supplements and herbs help?

• A magnesium deficiency increases circulating catecholamines, which is a mediator in platelet aggregation. The platelets in migraine sufferers show significant differences from normal platelets, both during and between attacks, and magnesium helps to normalise this.
• Calcium is good for muscle relaxation.
• Quercetin may help by inhibiting the pathways of inflammation.
• Niacin is a vasodilator and has been recommended in the treatment of migraines for a very long time; however, it may not be good for cluster headaches.
• Chromium helps to stabilise blood sugar levels if hypoglycaemia is suspected.
• Feverfew has shown to decrease the frequency and intensity of the attacks, especially in migraines. This is probably due to its ability to inhibit the secretion of serotonin from platelets, decrease blood vessels response to vasoconstrictors, and inhibit the production of inflammatory substances. This slows down the expansion of the blood vessels, preventing the throbbing head pain.
• Valeriana officinalis can help to reduce discomfort due to its sedative effect.
• White willow bark is a natural pain reliever.
• Skullcap and passionflower induce relaxation.
• Goldenseal helps to improve bowel function.
• Ginger helps to decrease inflammation in liver and stomach.
• Chamomile and rosemary teas are a good combination for headaches.
• Peppermint tea is good for headaches caused by indigestion.

How else can I improve my physical health?

Start a detox program. Always consult a naturopath or nutritionist first.

Hot and cold treatment (see **Therapies**), especially to skull, neck and shoulders, is useful to normalise circulation.

How can I improve my emotional, mental and spiritual health?

Set up a stress management programme.

Learn to say 'no' and take time out for yourself.

With the coaching programme release all negative emotions, limiting beliefs and pain held in the body, and do the exercises for forgiveness and solving difficult problems.

Practice daily meditation. This makes it virtually impossible for the body to develop non-serious recurring headaches.

When you have a headache it may be useful to give it a shape and a form. What does it look like? What is its highest purpose for you? What is it that it wants you to pay attention to, so that if you were to pay attention to it, the headache would disappear? Thank it for bringing all this to your awareness. Then keep on visualising your headache, put it in a frame, and shrink it down until it is as small as a tiny feather. Then blow it away, and watch it gently disappear from your life.

When should I contact a medical doctor?

• If you are vomiting and have a headache at the back of your head and you do not normally experience headaches.
• If lying down makes the headache worse, if it is worse in the morning, or if coughing and sneezing aggravate it.
• If you start to have personality changes
• If you experience weakness in your limbs
• If you have scalp tenderness and systemic symptoms (a general feeling of being unwell, low grade fever and malaise)
• If you have a severe headache, sensitivity to light, nausea, fever, neck stiffness and irritability.
• If you suffer confusion
• Unexplained episodes of fainting

Which therapies help for non-serious headaches and migraines?

Osteopathy and chiropractic help by releasing muscular and fascial tension and restoring proper joint movement in the neck, upper back, sacrum, ribs and the diaphragm.

Cranial osteopathy is particularly useful after whiplash injuries, migraines, falls to the sacrum, blows to the head, dental work and in the treatment of children

Tibetan, ayurvedic and Chinese medicine are highly beneficial through the use of herbs, massage and acupuncture.

Massage helps by releasing stress and tension in the muscles. It is especially useful in conjunction with osteopathy and chiropractic.

Alexander technique, yoga and Pilates help by aligning the musculo-skeletal framework and making you more aware of your posture.

NLP, hypnotherapy and well-being coaching help if the headache is of an emotional nature, because they assist you in releasing negative emotions and help you move forward with more appropriate strategies in place, so that your body does not need to develop a headache in order for you to stop and listen, or for you to be able to avoid a situation you do not want to deal with.

Homeopathy has many good remedies.

Healing helps to balance the emotions.

Useful affirmations

"Life is perfect just as it is."
"I relax and let go of everything I do not need, and welcome with joy those things that nourish me."

"I am perfect just as I am."

Heart Disease

Heart disease is the main killer in the western world and includes such diseases as angina (chest pain), arteriosclerosis (hardening of the arteries), atherosclerosis (hardening of the larger arteries such as the aorta, coronary and cerebral arteries), myocardial infarction (heart attack), stroke and congestive heart failure. The symptoms vary according to what structures are affected.

Angina

This may give a sensation of squeezing, crushing, burning, pressing, choking or aching in the chest. Sometimes pain may radiate to the arm (usually the left), neck, jaw, throat or shoulder blade. It can also present with a burning indigestion, nausea, shortness of breath and toothache. It is normally not a stabbing sensation and very rarely gives severe pain. It usually lasts for only a few minutes, and is typically precipitated by exertion, stress, anxiety or anger.

Atherosclerosis

Usually gives no symptoms until arteries are 90% blocked. The symptoms may vary according to the site of the main affected area:
• Angina for coronary arteries
• Intermittent and frequent leg cramps while walking, with relief of pain upon stopping
• Gradual deterioration of mental ability (cerebral vessels)
• Fatigue (lack of blood supply to the heart)
• Dizziness (lack of blood supply to the head and/or inner ears)
• Tinnitus (due to circulation to the inner ears)

Myocardial infarction

This is the development of ischaemia and necrosis of myocardial tissue, and is usually caused by narrowing of the coronary arteries, spasm of the coronary arteries, platelet aggregation and embolism, aortic stenosis, endocarditis, a thrombus secondary to rheumatic heart disease, or a thrombus on prosthetic mitral or aortic valve. It is characterised by extreme fatigue several days prior to the attack.

What are the signs and symptoms?

May give severe squeezing or crushing chest pain, which can radiate down both arms, as well as into the neck, jaw, throat and upper back. It can give a feeling of indigestion, and there may be nausea, pallor, loss of speech and/or vision, increased perspiration, shortness of breath, numbness, faintness and weakness. It can feel like a severe angina attack that lasts for longer than 30 minutes, and is unrelieved by rest or nitroglycerin.

Aneurysm

This is abnormal dilation in the wall of the artery or vein. It occurs when the vessel wall weakens from trauma, vascular disease, infection and atherosclerosis. It usually affects the aorta (thoracic or abdominal), popliteal and femoral arteries. An abdominal aneurysm may be asymptomatic (in 30–60%) until it ruptures (usually when it is wider than 5 cm), which quickly can lead to death.

What are the signs and symptoms?

Both an abdominal and a popliteal aneurysm can be felt as a pulsating mass (in the abdomen and behind the knee). An abdominal aneurysm may also give chest pain, dull ache in mid abdomen, groin and/or leg pain. When it has ruptured, it will give severe pain in the chest with a tearing sensation, and it may radiate to the neck, low back, shoulders and abdomen. There will be a palpable pulsating mass, increased pulse rate, decreased systemic blood pressure, light headedness, nausea, and asymmetry of the brachial, carotid and femoral pulses.

Stroke

This can be caused by a blood clot that dislodges from another part of the body (embolism) and is carried by the blood to the brain, a blood clot formed by the cerebral arteries in the brain, narrowing of the arteries (atherosclerosis) that strangulates the blood supply to the brain or a haemorrhage (rupture of blood vessels) in the brain.

Congestive heart failure

This can be either left ventricular failure (LVF) or right ventricular failure (RVF).

What causes LVF?

LVF is due to decreased cardiac output, which increases pulmonary venous pressure. This leads to increased pressure of left ventricle as blood accumulates there. In turn, the pressure in the left atrium increases, leading to a backlog of blood into the lungs resulting in pulmonary oedema and hypertension. It develops in coronary artery disease, aortic valve stenosis, hypertension and congenital defects, such as ventricular septal defect. It leads to changes in lungs, kidney and brain. Failure of one ventricle leads to failure of the other (ventricular interdependence), and often leads to RVF.

What causes RVF?

RVF is due to increased pressure in the right atrium, which leads to increased venous pres-

sure in the systemic circulation. This in turn leads to accumulation of fluid leading to oedema in the peripheral tissues and viscera. The jugular venous pressure is also increased. It develops in LVF, mitral and pulmonary stenosis, multiple pulmonary emboli, tricuspid regurgitation, right ventricular infarction and aortic septal defect. It leads to changes in the liver, spleen, subcutaneous and portal systems.

What are the risk factors?

Physical and emotional stress, pregnancy, dysrhythmia, fever, infection, anaemia, thyroid disorders, pulmonary disorders, Paget's disease, and some medications (leading to poor kidney function).

Signs and symptoms of LVF

- Shortness of breath and fatigue
- A persistent spasmodic cough on exertion
- Shortness of breath during the night and when lying down
- Increased heart beat
- Weight gain and oedema
- Muscle weakness
- Irritation and restlessness
- Decreased kidney function leading to increased urinary output

Signs and symptoms of RVF

- Increased fatigue
- Oedema that is symmetrical and begins in the ankles
- Pitting oedema (when a pressure mark is left on your skin after palpating it firmly)
- Oedema in the area of the sacrum and at the back of thighs
- Pain in the right upper abdomen
- Cyanosis (blue colour) of the nail beds
- Increased jugular venous pressure
- Systemic venous congestion leading to distortion of the neck veins

What are the general causes of heart disease?

• A diet rich in saturated fats, refined carbohydrates, overheated or oxidised vegetable oils, salt, sugar, coffee and alcohol
• Smoking increases risk of heart disease dramatically
• Genetic factors
• Stress and/or constant worrying
• 'Type A' personality, such as aggressiveness, impatience, competitiveness and always feeling time pressure
• Lack of exercise. This is partly because exercise improves the function of the heart and partly because it lowers the bad (LDL) cholesterol levels and increases the good (HDL) cholesterol levels. Exercise also decreases stress levels in the body by getting rid of excess adrenaline.
• Obesity
• Birth control pills, since they seem to increase cholesterol levels
• Soft water
• Various diseases, such as hypertension, diabetes and gout
• Certain drugs that increase cholesterol levels, such as some diuretics

Research has found that a deficiency in B6, folic acid and B12 can lead to increased homocysteinuria, which can increase the risk of heart disease (24). A study undertaken in 1995 showed that taking these supplements decreased the risk of developing heart disease (25).

Magnesium deficiency has been linked with increased risk of angina and heart disease (26). Magnesium deficiencies are common in patients with congestive heart failure, and low levels in these patients also reduce their chance of survival (27). Magnesium supplementation can help in patients with arrhythmia due to atrial fibrillation (28).

Many sufferers of heart disease are also deficient in Coenzyme Q10. Supplementation of CoQ10 has helped in patients with congestive heart failure (29,30) and in mitral valve prolapse and cardiomyopathy (31,32).

What are the psychosomatic causes?

In a psychosomatic context problems with the heart may relate to how we deal with the emotional aspects of ourselves. It may indicate lack of joy in our lives, stress, emotional instability, insecurity and/or placing too much importance on factors in our lives, which do not give lasting joy, such as status, money or power. It may also be due to an inability to stand up for oneself, set boundaries and being able to say 'no'. This leads to increased internal tension which places a heavy burden on the heart.

How can I help in regards to the diet?

• A vegetarian diet has shown to be protective against heart disease, therefore increase consumption of fruits and vegetables. Use olive oil in salads and food. Use butter sparingly instead of margarine (contains trans-fatty acids, which have been proven to worsen atherosclerosis).
• Eat plenty of coldwater fatty fish, such as mackerel, herring and salmon.
• Use onions freely in cooking, since they decrease platelet aggregation and decrease the risk of developing blood clots by inhibiting fibrin formation (component in clots).
• Hawthorn berries have a vasodilatory effect which decreases blood pressure and reduces angina. It is also effective in early stages of congestive heart failure (33) and minor arrhythmias.
• Alfalfa decreases blood cholesterol.
• Red grape juice is beneficial and in naturopathy it is regarded as an excellent blood cleanser.
• Take psyllium husks, oat bran and/or whole linseeds daily to improve the function of the digestive tract and avoid constipation. The fibre

binds to cholesterol and reduces the total cholesterol levels.

What should I avoid?

Avoid all refined, fried and fatty foods. Decrease consumption of animal fats, such as meat, cheese, full fat milk, ice cream, cream and butter. Avoid margarine, which contains trans-fatty acids (worsen atherosclerosis)

Which supplements and herbs help?

• A good multivitamin and mineral tablet is useful. Make sure it contains copper, since this mineral is often deficient in the western diet, which can contribute to an increase in cholesterol.

• Vitamin C with bioflavonoids decreases platelet aggregation

• Beta-carotene is a very potent antioxidant which helps to lower the free radicals in the body, thus helping to reduce the formation of atherosclerosis.

• Vitamin E increases circulation, decreases platelet aggregation and increases the good cholesterol (HDL) levels. If on blood thinning drugs do not take any extra vitamin E.

• B-complex helps in a variety of ways, since the various vitamins have different action. Some of them help in lowering the bad cholesterol (LDL) and reducing platelet aggregation. Folic acid acts as a vasodilator.

• Magnesium is very important and is often found to be deficient in people with heart disease. It helps to decrease platelet aggregation, decreases LDL and increases HDL and acts as a vasodilator. Too much vitamin D will lead to a deficiency in magnesium, and many drugs used for treating heart disease (diuretics, beta-blockers) lead to magnesium depletion.

• Coenzyme Q10 is an antioxidant and has been shown to strengthen the heart. It also aids in energy metabolism.

• Chromium may be needed since it is linked with diabetes, which can predispose to heart disease. Chromium levels decrease with age and the typical western diet is very low in chromium anyway due to the processed carbohydrates.

• Fish oil and flax seed oil supplements, since these fatty acids decrease cholesterols and platelet aggregation (when it sticks to the arterial walls).

• L-carnitine helps to stimulate the breakdown of fats, and is essential for the transport of fat into the cells. A deficiency in carnitine levels leads to reduced fatty acid circulation, which decreases energy production.

• Take garlic capsules daily and use lots of fresh garlic in cooking. It decreases cholesterol, blood viscosity and platelet aggregation.

• Ginger decreases platelet aggregation.

How else can I improve my physical health?

• Exercise daily, such as brisk walking and cycling. This improves the function of the heart and reduces amount of LDL cholesterol.

• Yoga and Pilates are beneficial, since a flexible, strong and balanced spine promotes a healthy nerve, blood and lymphatic function to all organs, including the heart.

• If you are overweight your heart has to work harder, so if needed take steps to lose weight.

How can I improve my emotional, mental and spiritual health?

Daily meditation is needed. This will reduce stress hormones in the body, lower blood pressure and reduce cholesterol levels.

Take it easier. Let go of being a perfectionist.

Deal with your emotions and avoid suppressing them. Negative emotions cause a stress response in the body, which increases the pressure on the cardiovascular system.

Learn to set boundaries and be able to say 'no'. Remember that 'no' is a complete sentence in itself. You do not have to give any reasons. Just a simple 'no' is enough.

With the aid of the coaching programme do the exercises for releasing negative emotions, releasing emotional pain held in the body (heart), reaching, forgiveness, solving difficult problems, and achieving your ideal day.

What gives you joy and pleasure? If you look at your day, week, month and year, how much of your time do you spend doing what you truly love doing? Which steps can you take to allow for more joy in your life?

How much joy and happiness do you give to others? How much joy and happiness do you allow others to give to you? Remember that what you give you receive, and what you receive you can give.

A good daily meditation is to sit still and go deep within. Place your awareness in your heart. Look inside your heart and just notice what it looks like. Is it healthy and happy? Or are there any dark areas, any sad and constricted places? When you find these areas go there and sink into them. Feel the feeling that is there, just allow it to come up. Then sink beneath that feeling to the next layer of emotion. Feel this one too, and keep doing this until you feel there are no more layers. Then sink beneath this final layer, because underneath it is always a positive layer. Usually it feels like love, joy, light or happiness. Stay there for a few moments. Then open up the top of your head and draw in universal love and send it into your heart. Keep sending this love until you feel your heart is completely healed. Then look around your heart again and notice how different it looks when it is healthy and happy.

Which therapies help?

Tibetan, ayurvedic and Chinese medicine help by restoring well-being within the cardio-vascular, digestive and nervous systems.

Osteopathy and chiropractic help by improving nerve and blood flow to the heart, by working on the upper neck, the upper thoracic spine, ribcage and clavicles. Cranial osteopathic techniques also help to balance the nervous system.

Reflexology, shiatzu and acupressure help by stimulating the cardio-vascular system, adrenal glands and digestive tract.

Healing helps by releasing negative emotions that restore the energy levels.

NLP, hypnotherapy and well-being coaching help by releasing past negative emotions and limiting beliefs.

Useful affirmations

"My heart is filled with love and joy."

"As I let go of the past I make room for joy and happiness to enter my life and heart."

"I am worthy of giving and receiving love, because I am an eternal being made of love."

Hyperactivity

True hyperactivity is a behavioural disorder, which is characterised by impulsiveness, inability to sit still, lack of co-ordination, emotional outbursts, poor memory, inability to concentrate for any length of time, short attention span and slow learning. Then there is what I refer to as 'slight hyperactivity', which is when a child has some of the symptoms above, but not to the severity of a true behavioural disorder.

What causes it?

The cause is largely unknown, but some factors seem to contribute, such as food additives and colourings, salicylates in foods, phosphate in processed and canned foods, allergies/sensitivities, nutritional deficiencies, emotional trauma and a difficult birth.

How can a difficult birth lead to a restless child?

A normal birth is one of the most strenuous experience of our lives, it has been estimated that the child produces enough stress hormones to potentially kill an adult. So when there is a difficult birth it can set up a highly charged central nervous system with the child being in a constant state of tension. It may then become difficult for the child to switch off and become settled. After a while this may become a pattern of behaviour.

How does diet play a role?

Food additives, colourings, artificial sweeteners, sugar and food sensitivities attack the healthy balance in the body, especially in children who are sensitive to such poison. Some children are more robust than others and show no obvious symptoms when eating such substances, although it certainly is not healthy. Others show violent signs, affecting their whole behaviour.

Deficiencies have been linked with hyperactivity, such as B6, iron, zinc, calcium, magnesium and essential fatty acids. Excess levels of copper affect moods, since copper inhibits enzyme production necessary for serotonin production. Excess of aluminum and lead have been linked with hyperactivity.

What are the psychosomatic causes?

Hyperactivity may be a way for the child to avoid dealing with his own circumstances and avoid feeling his deep emotions. This is not a conscious act, since children do not know how to voice their feelings. Instead the pressure builds up inside him and he acts out. It may be a way of getting attention, usually due to deep feelings of insecurity and vulnerability. Perhaps his circumstances are not very supportive; maybe he does not feel wanted and loved. It may be that the birth itself was so traumatic that the fear felt at that time was too much for him to cope with. Therefore he is constantly charging around to avoid feeling his deep fear, and his central nervous system may not be able to switch off.

How can I help in regards to the diet?

• Eat a healthy, organic diet made up of wholemeal unrefined foods, vegetables, and fruits low in salicylates (such as bananas, kiwi, pear and pineapple).
• Increase intake of seeds, such as sesame, sunflower and pumpkin. They are an excellent source of essential fatty acids as well as vitamins and minerals.
• Increase intake of pulses, lentils and fish (high protein content).
• Increase intake of foods high in iron, zinc, calcium and magnesium (see Therapies).
• Drink plenty of mineral water.

What should I avoid?

• Remove all additives, colourings, preservatives, pesticides, salt and sugar from the diet. Watch out for all artificial sweeteners. Of these, aspartame is the most common, and it has been shown to affect our nervous system negatively, in the form of depression, anxiety and headaches.
• There is also a connection between hyperactivity and refined sugar consumption.
• Avoid soft drinks, chocolate, colas and tea.
• Remove any known allergens or food sensitivities. (see **Food Allergies**).
• Remove all processed and canned foods as well as carbonated drinks, since these are high in phosphate, which can aggravate aggressive behaviour (34). Phosphate also makes calcium leach out of bones, which reduces bone density.

Many children have a salicylates sensitivity, so it is useful to avoid foods rich in natural salicylates such as almonds, apples, apricots, blackberries, grapes, cherries, clementines, cloves, cranberries, cucumber, nectarines, oranges, tangerines, mint, peaches, peppers, plums, prunes, raisins, raspberries, strawberries, tea and tomatoes.

Which supplements and herbs help?

• A good multivitamin and mineral supplement (free from sweeteners and colourings)
• Essential fatty acids, such as flaxseed oil (omega 3 and 6) and fish oil (omega 3)
• Chamomile and passionflower are calming on the central nervous system.

How else can I support my child's physical health?

Regular daily exercise is important. It should be vigourous enough to induce sweating. If your child likes any particular form of exercise or sport, then encourage it as much as possible.

Through exercising he will use up excess adrenaline and other stress hormones, which will allow his nervous system to calm down.

How can I help my child's emotional and mental health?

Think of your own actions in relation to your child. Remember he learns by copying you. If you remain calm and centered when you are under stress, you teach your child to do the same.

Think of the language you use and what internal representation you give your child. The brain can't compute a negative command. Therefore always say what you want him to do, rather than what you don't want him to do. For instance, if he is shouting at his brother, instead of saying, "Don't shout at your brother" say, "Speak calmly and nicely to your brother."

Listen to what you say to him. How often do you tell him how much you love him, what a good boy he is and how clever he is? How often do you tell him that he is annoying, that he is a bad boy and that he makes you really angry? How would you react if your parents said these different things to you? I am sure the first three would induce a sense of happiness within you and the latter three would cause you to feel bad about yourself. When you feel happy and loved you are more likely to co-operate, and when you feel bad you are more likely to lash out and react with anger.

Use positive reinforcement to encourage him to do something, instead of resorting to threats and punishments. For example, if he does not want to get dressed for school, instead of shouting at him and getting angry, try to make it into a game, such as "let's see if you can get dressed before I count to ten." Children love games, especially if they think they can win. By letting him get dressed before you reach the count of ten, you allow him to feel good about himself, and he is much more willing to do what you request of him.

Talk to him the way you want him to talk to you and others, using words that increase his self-esteem. If he does an inappropriate action, tell him calmly what you want him to do instead. When he does what you ask him to do, tell him what a good boy he is. This allows him to experience feeling good about himself instead of feeling bad when he is being told off.

Children respond very well to positive rewards. Keep a star-chart and tell your child what you want him to do; every time he does it he gets a star. After five or ten stars he gets a reward, such as special time with mummy or daddy or a present. You will be surprised how quickly he will want to do the tasks you set for him.

Take up yoga with your child. Make it into a fun game where you set aside time each week for the two of you (or perhaps the whole family) to do yoga together. Remember to reward him with a star afterwards for being so good.

It is highly useful for you to meditate daily, so that you remain calm and centred.

A good technique to use is to ask him, "If I had a magic wand, and you could wish for anything, what would you wish for?" and "If your Fairy Godmother/Magical Wizard was standing here in front of you and asked you what you needed from her/him in order for you to be happy and relaxed, what would you say?" You may be very surprised at the answers you get, because these questions engage the unconscious mind.

Make sure he spends time outdoors, because nature has a calming influence on the whole being.

Which therapies help?

Cranial osteopathy helps to balance the central nervous system, which often is taken into over-drive in hyperactive individuals. Some children who have had a difficult gestation or delivery (very fast, very long, assisted or caesarian) may be difficult to settle, be poor sleepers and have difficulty sitting still, which in turn may develop into constant fidgeting and hyperactivity. These children often have stresses and strains within their neuro-musculo-skeletal structure, which benefit greatly from treatment. It can also address an underlying middle ear problem, which could lead to decreased hearing, making learning, listening and concentration more difficult.

Acupuncture helps by addressing imbalances within the energy system in the body, as well as improving the gastro-intestinal system, so that nutrients are properly digested.

Kinesiology helps by establishing any food sensitivities and by balancing the neuro-musculo-skeletal system

Medical herbalism has many herbs which have a calming effect on the central nervous system.

Homeopathy has remedies which help to balance the emotions as well as the nervous system.

Healing is excellent for balancing the emotions and the energy levels in the body.

Bach flower remedies are often helpful.

NLP, hypnotherapy and well-being coaching help by releasing past negative emotions, limiting beliefs and by changing unwanted states and behaviours (for both the child and/or the parents). It also helps the child to come up with his own solutions for how he can do things differently.

Useful affirmations

"It is safe for me to relax."

"I enjoy the stillness within me."

"I am happy being me."

Hypertension

A normal blood pressure reading is 120/80. The systolic reading (120) shows the maximum pressure the heart is exerting during its contraction, whilst the lower reading is the diastolic pressure the heart is experiencing when it is resting between contractions. Mild hypertension ranges from 120–160/90–104, moderate hypertension from 140–180/105–114, and severe hypertension is 160/115 or above. Increased blood pressure correlates with an increased risk of having a heart attack or a stroke.

What are the two types of hypertension?

There is essential hypertension, which accounts for 90–95% of all cases, and secondary hypertension.
• Essential hypertension is usually due to a variety of factors, such as diet (high fat, salt and meat intake), stress, overweight, alcohol, coffee, smoking, lack of exercise, atherosclerosis, oral contraceptives, heavy metal exposure (cadmium and lead), and food allergies or sensitivities.
• Secondary hypertension is normally due to renal disease (kidneys), adrenal problems (adrenaline constricts the blood vessels), pregnancy (as in pre-eclampsia) and Cushing's syndrome.

What are the signs and symptoms?

Usually no signs are present, which make it so dangerous. If there are any signs they may include dizziness, headache, tiredness, insomnia, nose bleeds, breathing problems, nervousness, anxiety, irritability and gastrointestinal problems.

What are the psychosomatic causes?

Hypertension may be caused by repressed emotion, such as deep fear, anger and/or anxiety and the blood pressure rises from the sheer force of not letting these emotions come up to the surface.

What are the treatments for hypertension?

Mild hypertension responds very well to a change in diet, lifestyle and exercise. It is usually best to try to reduce a mild increase in blood pressure through natural means, since blood pressure lowering drugs have side effects, such as impotence, fatigue and headache.

How can I help in regards to my diet?

• Increase intake of vegetables, fruits and seeds (sunflower, pumpkin and sesame).
• Increase foods high in potassium such as bananas, avocados, melons, broccoli, potatoes, cauliflower and cabbage since these will help to balance the sodium in the body.
• Eat lots of garlic and onions. Both have shown to decrease blood pressure and to reduce cholesterol (55).
• Increase fibre consumption, such as linseeds, psyllium husks and oat fibre. This aids proper elimination and reduces the cholesterol in the blood, since cholesterol binds to the fibre in the gut and in this way is cleared from the body.
• To aid the function of the kidneys and liver drink diluted fresh juice of carrots, beetroots and lemons daily.

What should I avoid?

• It is absolutely necessary to reduce salt intake and use herbal seasoning instead. Do not eat tinned and processed foods since they have a high salt content.

• Reduce meat—preferably eliminate it totally.
• Decrease sugar and fat intake.
• Avoid caffeine (coffee, chocolate, cola drinks), since these increase the adrenal output.
• It is absolutely essential to stop smoking.

Which supplements and herbs help?

• Magnesium and calcium help to decrease blood pressure so increase consumption of foods high in these such as nuts, green leafy vegetables and soya beans. If needed take supplements.
• Hawthorn berries have a mild effect on reducing blood pressure. They also increase the intracellular vitamin C levels, strengthen the capillaries, and help in reducing the deposition of cholesterol in arterial walls.
• Vitamin C is beneficial. Studies have shown that the higher the intake of vitamin C the lower the blood pressure (56). It also helps to strengthen the walls of the capillaries. In individuals with lead poisoning, vitamin C helps to excrete lead from the body.
• Essential fatty acids such as in olive oil, flax seed oil and fish oil are very effective in lowering blood pressure (57,58).
• Coenzyme Q10 helps since people with hypertension are often deficient in CoQ10. It aids metabolism and heart function and has a blood pressure lowering effect (59).

How else can I improve my physical health?

• Lose weight if necessary.
• Daily exercise, deep breathing and skin brushing help detoxify the liver and help the body get rid of excess adrenaline.

How can I improve my emotional, mental and spiritual health?

Learn to say 'no' and to prioritise. Find the triggers that increase your internal stress, and do something about them.

With the coaching programme release all negative emotions, limiting beliefs and do the exercises for forgiveness and for solving difficult problems. This releases tension from your body and mind.

What are the lessons for you from having hypertension in your life? What does it need you to pay attention to, know or learn, for it to disappear?

Practice meditation and breathing exercise daily. This will balance your central nervous system and lower your blood pressure.

Write a gratitude journal every day before going to bed. This trains your mind to focus on all the positive aspects of your life.

Which therapies help?

Tibetan, ayurvedic and Chinese medicine help to balance the central nervous system and aid the function of the heart.

Reflexology, acupressure and shiatzu help by stimulating pressure points related to the cardio-vascular system and nervous system.

Healing helps by releasing built up tension, balancing the emotions and restoring energy.

Homeopathy has many suitable remedies.

Osteopathy, cranial osteopathy and chiropractic help by improving the function of the cardio-vascular system and by balancing the central nervous system.

NLP, hypnotherapy and well-being coaching help to release negative emotions and change unwanted states and behaviours.

Useful affirmations

"I release the old and embrace the new with peace and love."

"My heart is filled with love and for every heartbeat this love flows to every cell of my being."

Hypoglycaemia

This is a condition where blood glucose levels are lower than normal due to a defect in carbohydrate metabolism. Hypoglycaemia is very common in the western world, and even though it is not a disease, it shows that there is a dysfunction in the working of many glands and organs.

What are the signs and symptoms?

Irritability, nervousness, anxiety, depression, crying, headaches, fatigue, dizziness, poor concentration, trembling, fainting, double vision and hyperactivity.

If these symptoms are worse three to four hours after a meal, and disappear when eating, it is very likely hypoglycaemia. Often extreme tiredness can be felt an hour after eating.

What causes it?

• A diet made up of an excess of refined carbohydrates, which will be easily converted to glucose in the body, forcing the pancreas to secrete big doses of insulin to help clear this from the blood. This will then lead to a drastic fall in blood sugar levels, giving rise to the above mentioned symptoms.
• Stress will lead to an overproduction of adrenaline, since the body is preparing for a fight or flight situation. The adrenaline converts stored glycogen in the liver and muscle tissue and releases this into the blood stream to give more energy to the body in case it needs to fight or flee. When this does not happen the pancreas needs to secrete insulin to clear the glucose from the blood, since blood glucose levels need to be within a very tight range for normal brain function.
• Caffeine stimulates the adrenal glands to secrete adrenaline, which is why you feel more energetic after drinking coffee or cola, but it also sets up the same viscous cycle as described above.
• Large meals, since this increases the workload of the pancreas.
• Not eating regularly.
• Excessive exercise.
• Alcohol and/or drug abuse. Alcohol contains high quantities of sugar, which will again lead to an increased production of insulin. Alcohol and drugs damage the liver, which increases the strain on the pancreas.
• Smoking alters blood sugar levels.
• Diabetes can often cause hypoglycaemic episodes, since the body has difficulty regulating its own blood sugar efficiently.
• Pregnancy
• Candida
• Hypothyroidism, tumour of the pancreas and a dysfunctional pituitary.

What about the psychosomatic causes?

In a psychosomatic context hypoglycaemia may be an indication of an individual who is giving too much, and not nourishing the self enough. It may also reflect an individual who is subjected to a lot of emotional and mental stress, which causes the adrenal glands to become hyperactive, thereby releasing blood sugar into the blood at such a pace that the pancreas has to secrete large amounts of insulin to clear it, which leads to a rapid drop in blood sugar levels.

How can I help in regards to the diet?

• Eat small, frequent, regular meals to decrease stress on the pancreas and adrenal glands.
• Eat whole grains, nuts, seeds, brown bread, brown pasta, brown rice, fish, chicken and vegetables.
• Eat fruit in moderation and it may help to combine it with some yoghurt or nuts.

However, fructose (sugar found in fruit) produces less sharp blood sugar elevation than starch and may increase the body's sensitivity to insulin (60,61). Therefore if you do not react negatively when you eat fruit, then you can probably consume it regularly.

What should I avoid?

Avoid all sugar, soft drinks, sweets, cakes, biscuits, white bread, white pasta and white rice, since these are refined carbohydrates and therefore convert to glucose too quickly.

Which supplements and herbs help?

• Vitamin C with bioflavonoids is important to alleviate the burden on the adrenal glands, as well as helping the efficiency of the insulin.
• B-complex is needed for proper functioning of carbohydrate metabolism.
• Zinc is needed for insulin production as well as helping to combat the side effects of stress.
• Magnesium can help to regulate both insulin and blood sugar levels.
• Chromium helps to increase the glucose clearing activity of insulin. 200 micrograms per day is often recommended.
• Spirulina may help to normalise blood glucose levels.

How else can I improve my physical health?

Regular gentle cardiovascular exercise will help the body maintaining a healthy blood sugar balance.

Yoga and Pilates help to balance the whole body and mind, which both decrease stress levels and improve spinal mobility, thereby having a beneficial effect on the whole glandular system.

How can I improve my emotional, mental and spiritual health?

Practice meditation and breathing exercises daily. This will calm your nervous system, balance your emotions and still your mind.

How much self-love are you practising? Do you constantly prioritise the needs of others before your own? Are your days filled with duties and obligations? Look at these questions, because the answers hold the key to how much love you show yourself. Remember that you can only give to others that which you have first given to yourself. Practising being loving to self means there is even more love within you to share with the rest of the world.

Look at all your personal, family and work relationships. Are they happy and fulfilling? Are they balanced and based on mutual respect and love? If they are not, then release whatever limiting beliefs and negative emotions you have formed, which are stopping you from experiencing harmony within all areas of your life. Everything starts in the mind, so when you change on the inside, your outside reality will change as well.

Visualise yourself in perfect health. Then send your pancreas, adrenal glands and blood as much love as you possibly can. Ask them when you decided to create your hypoglycaemia and for what purpose? Ask what your hypoglycaemia needs you to do, pay attention to or learn, in order for it to get better? Then act on this guidance.

Which therapies help?

Tibetan, ayurvedic and Chinese medicine and acupuncture are highly effective treatments for helping to restore health and function of the pancreas, liver, kidneys, adrenal glands and digestive tract.

Osteopathic and chiropractic treatment help by improving the function of the pancreas, kidneys, liver, gastrointestinal tract and adrenal glands by improving the nerve, blood and lymphatic flow. Cranial osteopathic techniques aid in balancing the central nervous system, thereby reducing the adrenaline output in the body.

Reflexology, shiatzu and acupressure help by balancing the pancreas, liver, adrenal glands and digestive tract through pressure points.

Healing is beneficial, both by working directly on the pancreas and adrenal glands, but also by working on the emotional stress within the body and mind.

Pilates helps by improving strength, flexibility and balance within the neuro-musculo-skeletal system, which helps to improve and normalise nerve and blood flow to all the abdominal organs.

Useful affirmations

"My life is filled with a constant source of sweetness and joy."

"I give and receive love easily and effortlessly."
" As I relax and trust life everything falls into place. All I have to do is keep being relaxed and trusting."

"It is my birthright to be happy. Therefore it is my birthright to fill my days with activities I love doing ."

Immune system

The immune system is a vital part of our protection from infectious disease and prevents tissues from becoming non-self tissues, such as cancers and tumours. It is one of the most complex and fascinating systems of the human body and has only fairly recently been understood by scientists and physicians.

What does the immune system consist of?

It consists of the lymphatic vessels and organs, such as the thymus, spleen, tonsils, adenoids, lymph nodes and various types of white cells, which engulf and destroy foreign particles, such as bacteria and initiates anti-body production to de-activate them. The liver also plays a role, because it produces the majority of lymph in the body, and houses special types of macrophages, which the integrity of the lymphatic system is highly dependent on.

What causes a low immune system?

• Undernourishment from malnutrition as seen in many third world countries, and vitamin deficiency as seen in many developing countries, where many eat a nutritionally poor, refined diet, high in fat, salt and additives. High intake of barbecued and smoked food can also strain the immune system (high in carcinogens).
• Too much sugar—in the form of glucose, fructose, sucrose, honey and various fruit juices—reduces the ability of the immune system to destroy bacteria for up to five hours. Sugar also competes with vitamin C for membrane transport sites, which makes it more difficult for the body to utilise vitamin C.
• Insufficient protein in the diet seems to reduce cell-mediated immunity and usually accompanies other nutrient deficiencies.

• Obesity, possibly due to elevated lipid and cholesterol levels and increased strain on heart, lungs and joints can contribute to a low immune system.

• Low levels of vitamin A have shown to decrease immune function and increase death rate in children suffering from a viral infection, such as measles. Supplementation of vitamin A in babies suffering from measles has shown to reduce the mortality rate (35).

• Environmental chemicals and heavy metals cause a lowered immune system.

• Alcohol consumption. Impairment of alcohol on the immune system is in direct proportion to the amount of alcohol consumed (36).

• Stress increases levels of adrenaline and cortico-steroids, which release stored glucose from muscle tissue thereby increasing blood sugar, leading to the same problems as a diet high in sugar. It inhibits white blood cell function and formation and also causes the thymus gland to shrink. The greater the stress, the greater the damage to the immune system (37).

• Caffeine intake also increases adrenaline output.

• Other causes are food sensitivities, tobacco, sleep deprivation, depression, lack of social support, excessive exercise, repeated use of antibiotics, digestive tract disorders (poor absorption), chemotherapy and radiation.

What are the psychosomatic causes?

A low immune system may indicate an individual who is under some form of stress. Our immune system is closely linked to our stress response in the body, and an excess of stress, or prolonged stress, causes our bodies to wear out prematurely. Our brain and emotional states are also inseparable from our immune system, which is why negative thinking can make us ill, and positive thinking can make us well.

How can I help in regards to my diet?

Eat a healthy, organic diet, with plenty of fruits and vegetables and drink plenty of filtered water.

What should I avoid?

• Refined foods, sugar, salt, additives, artificial sweeteners, dairy products and red meat
• Avoid undiluted juices and soft drinks
• Avoid alcohol, caffeine, and tobacco
• Avoid any known food allergies/sensitivities

What should I do when I have an infection?

• Drink herbal teas, water and diluted fruit juices. Undiluted juices are high in fruit sugar, which reduces the white blood cell count and leaves the immune system weakened.

• Sleep, because during sleep the parasympathetic nervous system is at work and many immune enhancing functions take place.

• Do not suppress a fever unless it is above 104 degrees F (40 degrees C). A fever is the body's own natural immune response in dealing with an infection.

• Breathing exercises stimulate the lymphatics

• Stimulate the thymus gland (lower part of throat/upper chest) by doing hot and cold treatment (see **Therapies**).

• Do not exercise at all.

Which supplements and herbs help?

• Take echinacea three times a day at the onset of a cold, flu or an infection.

• Goldenseal and astralgus are good antiviral herbs.

• Zinc, propolis, vitamin C with bioflavonoids and vitamin A help the immune system. Zinc is needed for functioning of white blood cells and the thymus, and it inhibits growth of many viruses. Vitamin C helps fight viral infections and cancer by increasing interferon levels. It increases the hormone secretions by the thymus, enhancing it's function. It also helps white blood cell function and response. Vitamin C is often depleted during stress, because adrenaline needs vitamin C for its transport to body tissues, thereby reducing the amount of vitamin C available in the body.

• Eat plenty of garlic and try to increase consumption of ginger, sage, thyme and rosemary.

How can I improve my immune system?

• Take acidophilus daily to maintain healthy gut flora.
• Increase foods rich in B-vitamins, vitamin C, carotenes, vitamin E, selenium and essential fatty acids. B6 is needed for cell-mediated immunity and a lack of folic acid and B12 can cause a reduction of white blood cell production, decrease the function of white blood cells and reduce the size of the thymus. Carotenes are excellent antioxidants, which help the function of the thymus, since it is easily damaged by free radicals. Carotenes also help the immune system by increasing the number of helper T cells (38). Vitamin E and selenium help the function of white blood cells and of the thymus. Supplementation of vitamin E seems to increase T cell function (39). Iron deficiency can decrease immune function and is fairly common in children, menstruating women, and people with bleeding ulcers or who are taking aspirin daily. A supplement containing iron may be needed, but it should not be taken during an infection (except in chronic infections), since the body's natural response to an infection is to decrease the iron levels, because bacteria needs iron too.
• Take garlic capsules daily.
• If you are pregnant don't take vitamin A.
• It may be worth taking vitamin and mineral supplements if you are elderly or come down with infections regularly.

How can breast-feeding benefit a baby?

Research has shown that babies who have been exclusively breastfed for four months, have a thymus gland about twenty times bigger than non-breastfed babies (40). It also improves the bonding between mother and child.

How else can I improve my physical health?

Regular, moderate exercise which activates deep diaphragmatic breathing, increases the lymphatic function, which helps the body to eliminate waste products. A great lymphatic pumping exercise is to go up on to your tiptoes while swinging your arms back, then as you lower your heels, bring your arms forward. Breathe out vigourously as you go up on to your tiptoes and breathe out as you go down. Do this for a few minutes.

Daily breathing exercises are recommended.

Pilates and yoga are great forms of exercises.

Stimulate your lymphatic system daily by brushing your skin with a loofah. Brush with small circular motions starting at the end of your limbs and moving up towards the heart.

After a warm shower, finish with ice-cold water to enhance your circulation.

How can I improve my emotional, mental and spiritual health?

Practice meditation regularly and do the exercises in the coaching programme for releasing negative emotions, limiting beliefs, forgiveness and solving difficult problems.

Visualise drawing a golden, healing light to you. Let it surround your body, and then allow it to enter through the top of your head. From your head let it flow down your spine, and into every cell of your being, bringing about a complete rejuvenation.

Listen to your body. What does it need from you in order to become well again? What does it want you to pay attention to? Listen to the answers and then act on them.

Develop an optimistic attitude towards life. Research has shown that this actually promotes health. So look for the positive in every situation in your life.

Which therapies help?

Tibetan, ayurvedic and Chinese medicine help by improving the immune system with the use of herbs, massage and acupuncture.

Medical herbalism has several useful herbs, such as echinacea and goldenseal.

Reflexology, shiatzu and acupressure help through stimulating pressure points related to the function of the immune system.

Healing helps to balance the emotions and to restore your energy levels.

Osteopathy and chiropractic help the immune system by promoting proper nerve, blood and lymphatic function, which enhance the general health of the body tissues.

Hypnotherapy, NLP and well-being coaching help by releasing negative emotions and limiting beliefs, which may have created an enormous amount of inner tension, depleting the immune system.

useful affirmations

"My mind and body are filled with peace."

"I have all the energy I need to heal this within me."

"I love my body and I am now able to give it what it needs."

Insomnia

Insomnia is very common and usually presents itself as a difficulty with falling asleep (sleep onset insomnia), or as frequent episodes of waking during the night or very early awakening (maintenance insomnia). It affects most people at some stage in their lives, usually at times of great stress. For some, their high levels of stress have become a 'normal' state of being, and they find it extremely difficult to switch off at night. Their minds are constantly racing, not knowing how to stop. Sleep is essential to our well-being, and without it we become irritable, aggressive, depressed and more prone to infections due to a lowered immune system.

What causes it?

There are many causes of insomnia with stress and psychological factors being the most common ones, but it can also be brought on by anxiety and depression (both forms of stress), drug and/or alcohol abuse, large caffeine consumption, poor diet leading to nutrient deficiencies (especially B-vitamins, calcium, magnesium), hypoglycaemia, allergies, food additives/colourings, heavy metal poisoning, electromagnetic disturbance, smoking, physical pain, hypo and hyperthyroidism, menopause, irregular sleeping hours and various medications, such as the birth control pill and beta-blockers.

What are the psychosomatic causes?

In a psychosomatic context insomnia may indicate an unwillingness to let go and trust life. When we are asleep our conscious minds must surrender to our unconscious minds, and if we are not willing, or able to do this due to fear, anxiety, stress, or tension, then insomnia will be the inevitable result. It is important to learn that we cannot always be in control, that it is necessary to let go of that control, and to trust that life will take care of itself. This is a vital aspect of health, the learning to let go...so many of us have lost this ability.

How can I help in regards to the diet?

Avoid all caffeinated drinks and food, such as coffee, tea, chocolate and cola. Caffeine increases the adrenaline production in the body, making you ready for a fight or flight episode. It also overcharges your sympathetic nervous system making it very difficult for you to get to sleep, since that is something that is done by the parasympathetic nervous system, which has been shut down by all the adrenaline. Adrenaline also increases the conversion of glucose from the muscles, making you ready to fight or flee, but since you probably end up doing neither, your blood sugar levels increase instead, which means your pancreas has to work harder producing insulin to clear the sugar away from the blood, leading to a fall in sugar levels.

For the same reason avoid refined carbohydrates, such as cakes, sweets and biscuits, since these will give a quick rise in blood sugar, followed by a sharp drop. The brain needs a constant supply of glucose (sugar) to function properly, and a drop in sugar levels alerts the brain that it needs more food, which means that you will wake up. Therefore never eat anything sweet just before going to bed, especially if you are prone to blood sugar swings.

Avoid all food that you know you have an allergy/sensitivity to, since it increases heart rate, and histamine release can alter sleep patterns, by altering the brain chemistry.

Avoid all drugs and alcohol. Alcohol increases adrenaline production in the body, and it also impairs tryptophan transport, which reduces levels of serotonin in the brain, which in turn impairs sleep.

How else can I improve my physical health?

Check for any thyroid or other endocrine problems.

It is important to get regular day light for the biological rhythm to function properly.

Exercise has been shown to increase general well-being and to improve the quality of sleep. It has also been found to decrease stress and depression, probably by releasing the build up of tension within the physical structure, therefore improving the health of both body and mind.

Avoid unnecessary exposure to electromagnetic fields, so avoid electric blankets, TV in bedrooms, and power lines.

Warm baths before bedtime can be helpful.

Which supplements and herbs help?

Supplement with a B-complex, calcium and magnesium 30-60 minutes before bedtime. This will help to relax the muscles and nerves. (A hot soya drink enriched with calcium is useful, since soya is high in magnesium).

Lavender and roman chamomile oil is relaxing. If you are not pregnant or taking any medication it may help to put a few drops in the bath, on a pillow or in a burner. Various herbs can be of help, such as chamomile, valerian and passion flower. These are very good as a tea in the evening to aid relaxation.

How can I improve my emotional, mental and spiritual health?

Regular meditation and breathing exercises are of utmost importance as this effectively reduces tension within the body-mind structure.

With the coaching programme release all negative emotions and limiting beliefs and do the exercises for forgiveness and solving difficult problems.

Relax and trust that life brings you everything you need. Practice seeing the lesson in every experience you have. Once you get the lesson all negative emotions associated with the experience disappears, and all you are left with are joy and wisdom.

Is it not true that in the end you can always learn something positive from everything that has ever happened, is happening and will ever happen to you in your life?

Be kind to yourself and do something every week, which brings you happiness.

Learn to say no and set your boundaries. Only take on tasks that you truly want to do, and let go of the rest.

You are only responsible for your own well-being and happiness, so only you have the power to change and create the life you want.

Which complementary treatments help?

Tibetan, ayurvedic and Chinese medicine and acupuncture help greatly to balance the nervous system and the mind.

Cranial osteopathy helps to balance the nervous system so it is not constantly overcharged.

Medical herbalism has many useful herbs.

Healing helps to balance the mind and body.

Useful affirmations

"I relax and trust that life brings me all that I need."

"For each breath I breathe in peace and calm."

Multiple Sclerosis

This is a progressive, degenerative disease of the central nervous system. It is caused by a gradual loss of the myelin sheaths (demyelination) covering the nerve cells in the brain and spinal cord. The myelin sheath helps to facilitate transmission of the nerve impulse, therefore without the myelin sheath the nerve function is lost.

What is it characterised by?

Periods of exacerbation and remission, where the symptoms vary depending on where the demyelination is occurring.

Who is affected?

Slightly more women than men are affected, and the onset is usually between 20-40 years. It is very rare after the age of 50. There seems to be a geographical predisposition for developing the disease. The areas of highest frequency rates are all located in the higher latitudes, both in the northern and southern hemispheres, such as Scandinavia, northern Europe, United Kingdom, New Zealand, Tasmania, United States and Canada. However, it is uncommon in Japan. It also appears to be of importance at what age one lives in any of these affected regions, since it seems to affect those who lives there for the first 15 years of their lives. If they move before the age of 15 to an area of low risk, their risk factor is reduced, whilst if they move in to a high risk area from a low risk area after the age of 15, there seems to be no increase in risk factor for developing the disease.

What are the signs and symptoms?

It is difficult to diagnose MS at its early stages, because the symptoms may vary so much.

Most commonly it affects the *motor function*, such as an increased tendency to drop things, clumsiness, weakness, a feeling of having a heavy limb or that a leg drags while walking.

The second most common finding is that it affects the *visual function*, and this can lead to symptoms such as blurred vision, double vision, blindness, and/or severe eyeball pain.

It can also affect other parts of the central nervous system, such as:
• the *sensory function*, which may give rise to pins and needles, numbness, dead feeling, or a tight sensation.
• the *vestibular function*, which may give rise to feelings of being light-headed or drunk, sensation of spinning, as well as nausea and/or vomiting.
• the *genito-urinary function*, which may give rise to incontinence, loss of feeling when bladder is full and/or loss of sexual function.

How is it diagnosed?

Certain tests can be done to help build up a picture, which can assist the specialist in making a diagnosis of MS. These include screening the CSF (cerebrospinal fluid) for raised IgG antibodies, since these are elevated in 80-90% of patients with MS. Nerve function tests can also be performed, and they can show abnormalities in most patients (94%) with established MS and in 67% of patients with suspected MS. However, these tests are not just positive in MS, but also in other neurological conditions that can mimic the signs and symptoms of MS. MRI scanning can also help to show any signs of demyelination.

What causes the demyelination?

The cause to MS has not conclusively been identified, but there seems to be a favour for the theory that it is an auto immune disease, and that several factors are contributing to the development and the severity of the progression of MS. These factors include the following;
• There is a strong link with MS and a diet rich in saturated fatty acids and animal fats. One of the first studies of this took place in Norway, where it was observed that inland farming communities had a much higher incidence of MS, than coastal fishing communities (62). The farmers diet was much higher in saturated fatty acids and animal fats, while the people that lived near the coast line ate more cold water fish, which are rich in poly unsaturated fatty acids. In Japan, where MS is very rare (despite being at a high latitude), the diet consists of large quantities of fish, sea food, seeds and soya, all very rich in polyunsaturated fatty acids.
• Some theories suggest that food allergies can aggravate MS, especially dairy and gluten, but also eggs. Areas with a high incidence of MS eat a diet rich in gluten and saturated fats, such as dairy.
• Many MS patients have found to be lacking in an antioxidant enzyme, GSH-Px, which is needed for cell protection from free-radical damage. Its decreased levels may make the myelin sheaths more open to damage (this may be due to genetic factors). This enzyme is found in two forms, selenium dependent and non-selenium dependent.
• In naturopathic and ayurvedic medicine toxicity is a common contributor to ill health. Toxicity can be due to a variety of factors, such as heavy metals, environmental toxins, food pesticides, additives, colourings, poor diet, alcohol, coffee, tea, cleaning chemicals, permanents and hair dyes. Therefore the individual would eliminate all aggravating factors and do a detox.

What about any psychosomatic causes?

MS can be an indication of an individual who is unconsciously inflamed with anger. This anger is so deep that is starts to affect the whole nervous system, which is the part of our being that controls all our functions, and our ability to experience life fully. It is as if we slowly create a prison around ourselves, so that we do not have to deal with and take responsibility for this inner anger. This can make us inflexible and rigid in our approach to ourselves, others and the world. It can also be an indication of someone who is refusing to stop and rest, even when the body and mind are crying out for it. Instead they carry on, refusing to accept help from anyone, while inside the resentment and anger builds up.

How can I help in regards to the diet?

• Eat organic as much as possible.
• Eat plenty of cold water fish (salmon, mackerel, herring), legumes, seeds (sunflower especially), soya, vegetables and fruits.
• Use cold pressed unsaturated oils on salads and in cooking.

What should I avoid?

• Avoid all refined foods, such as white flour, white rice, white sugar, white salt. Also avoid coffee, tea, cola and alcohol.
• If a sensitivity to any particular food substance has been noted, it should be eliminated from the diet. Common culprits are dairy, gluten (especially wheat), and citrus.
• Cut out completely all saturated fats, such as dairy (milk, butter, cream, ice-cream, cheese, yoghurt, creme fraiche), margarine, and all hydrogenated oils.
• Avoid meat, eggs and other animal foods (except the above mentioned fish).

Which supplements and herbs help?

• Supplement the diet with cod liver oil (omega 3) and flax seed oil (omega 3 and omega 6).

• With an increased consumption of polyunsaturated fatty acids it is important to also supplement with vitamin E, since the requirement for this vitamin then is increased. Selenium is needed too, since it may help to increase GSH-Px levels. Vitamin E also helps the body to utilise selenium better.
• Antioxidants (A, C and E) may be beneficial to help reduce the free-radicals in the body.
• A good B-complex, especially with B12, is important for proper nerve function. (A deficiency in B12 may aggravate MS).
• Take a good multivitamin and mineral tablet.
• Pancreatic enzymes to aid digestion have been shown to reduce severity and symptoms of demyelination affecting the sensory and visual function, as well as urinary and intestinal function.
• Ginkgo biloba may be useful as an antioxidant. It improves the blood flow to the nervous system and may help to enhance cell function. See a medical herbalist for advice.

How can I improve my physical health?

• Periods of detox fasting may be beneficial, but should only be done under strict supervision.
• Hot and cold showers help to stimulate circulation and aid elimination.
• Plenty of aerobic exercise. What type depends on individual ability.
• Avoid chemicals in make-up, hair and skin products.

How can I improve my emotional, mental and spiritual health?

• Meditation, visualisation and relaxation exercises are of utmost importance.
• Learn to let go of your anger. When you are angry with someone you only cut the wound within yourself deeper and deeper. Good exercises to do are "Release a negative emotion" and the "Forgiveness" meditations.

• Good daily mediation to release a negative emotion is the following: sit comfortably and feel how you drain all your anger away from your spirit, mind and body through the soles of your feet. Collect all your anger into a ball on the ground, then place this ball on a fire, and see how the blue-white heat from the fire purifies and cleanses your anger until it is all gone. Then a positive emotion rises from the fire, which will help you on your path in life. Breathe in this positive emotion. Let it fill your lungs, and as you breathe out send this positive emotion to every cell of your being—body, mind and spirit. Then do the same with any other negative emotions you may have.

• How much self-love do you practice? How much of your time do you fill with activities you love doing? Which steps can you take to ensure you create the balanced life you truly want from the bottom of your heart?

Which therapies help?

Tibetan, ayurvedic and Chinese medicine help by improving the function of the nervous and digestive systems,

Cranial osteopathy helps bring the central nervous system, and especially the CSF, into a better state of balance and health.

Massage helps relieve tired and strained muscles.

Kinesiology helps by balancing the energy and musculo-skeletal systems, and identifying any food allergens.

Medical herbalism helps through a variety of herbs. See a practitioner for advice.

Healing helps by balancing the emotions and restoring energy.

NLP, hypnotherapy and well-being coaching help by changing unwanted states and behaviours and by releasing negative emotions and limiting beliefs.

Useful affirmations

"As I forgive others I set myself free."

"It is now safe for me to let go of any negative emotion. As I do so I free myself to feel my own inner happiness."

"I now choose to experience a loving and happy world. I do so by choosing loving and happy thoughts."

Neck Pain

Neck pain is very common and nearly everyone experiences it at some stage in his or her life. It can be anything from a mild strain to a severe, agonising pain when it is difficult to lift the head up from the pillow, turn the head or chew food. It may also be accompanied by headache, dizziness, pain down one or both arms, pins and needles, numbness, muscle weakness and shooting pain along the course of a nerve.

Why is it so painful?

When there is a strain or injury to a body structure, such as the joints, tendons or muscles, histamine and other chemicals are released by the damaged tissue. This sets up an inflammatory reaction leading to swelling which increases the pressure on nearby structures causing pain. The chemicals also stimulate the nerves that transmit pain. This is the body's response to protect you from aggravating the injury, by making you stiffen up and feel pain as you place more strain on the injured area. Unfortunately it also restricts circulation which hinders important nutrients needed for healing from reaching the area. Appropriate treatment, such as osteopathy and chiropractic, decreases this reaction, speeds up the healing and allows the injured area to return to normal as quickly as possible.

What are the causes of neck pain?

There are many causes, since nearly every movement we do involves the neck. It is the first area of our body we gain control over as babies, and it is a highly important area for the function of our breathing, digestive system and central nervous system. Common causes of neck pain are:

• Neck joint restrictions, facet lock (the joint cannot move), or strain of the ligaments and muscles
• Whiplash injuries
• Prolapsed disc (usually only seen in trauma)
• Cervical spondylosis (osteoarthritis in the neck)
• Cervical rib syndrome
• Thoracic outlet syndrome

Other less common causes are:
• Cervical cord compression from a central disc protrusion or osteophyte formation
• Inflammatory conditions, such as rheumatoid arthritis and ankylosing spondylitis
• Infections, such as tuberculosis bacteria (TB) or vertebrae osteomyelitis
• Tumours
• Endocrine changes
• Psychological

What are the psychosomatic causes?

In a psychosomatic context neck pain may be an indication of a need to close off from the world, to retreat into one's own shell because the demands of life are just too much to bear. It may indicate a person who just grits his teeth and carries on during stress and conflict, regardless of the needs of others and/or of the self. Perhaps someone in the affected individual's life is literally being a 'pain in the neck'.

What can I do myself to help?

This will vary according to what is causing the pain. For arthritic conditions see Osteoarthritis or Rheumatoid Arthritis. For neck joint restrictions, facet locks and myoligamentous strain, see below:

Drink plenty of water and eat lots of fruits and vegetables, which contain vitamin C with bioflavonoids. This is necessary for the body in its healing process.

When the injury is acute, ice the area for 5–10 minutes at a time to decrease any inflammation. Rest as much as you can in a pain free position.

When the injury is sub-acute or even chronic, try hot and cold hydrotherapy (see Therapies). If at any time the heat seems to aggravate the injury, go back to the ice pack. Ice brings down the inflammation, heat aggravates it. Heat will relax the muscles, so you might feel better for a little while until the inflammation builds up again and the pain comes back with a vengeance. Alternating hot and cold will increase the circulation, which will speed up the recovery, but it can only do so when the inflammation has sufficiently subsided.

What should I avoid doing?

• Avoid painkillers. They cut off the pain signals reaching the brain, but the pain is there for a reason—to protect you from further damage. Some painkillers are anti-inflammatory, which is fine, but the ice pack is going to have an even more beneficial effect. If you have to take painkillers, do it sensibly and realise that you are still injured, even when the pain subsides.
• Avoid coffee, tea, chocolate, sugar and alcohol
• Avoid carrying anything heavy, such as groceries, a toddler, a rucksack or a briefcase
• Avoid sleeping on your stomach (strains neck)
• Avoid slumping

• Avoid wearing high-heeled shoes
• Avoid breaststroke swimming
• Avoid stress

Which supplements and herbs may be of help?

• Chamomile, skullcap, passionflower and valerian are natural herbal relaxants.
• White willow bark is a natural pain reliever.
• Proteolytic enzymes help with inflammation.
• Garlic helps to strengthen your immune system and fight against infection.

How can I improve my emotional, mental and spiritual health?

If you are someone who feels you must 'do it all yourself' or 'grin and bear it' or you are allowing someone else to really get to you, you must learn to say 'no'. You are only responsible for your own health and well-being, not for anyone else's. If you allow others to rely on you too much, you have to learn to set your boundaries, so that you only take on what you feel you can easily and effortlessly handle with joy.

What do you love filling your day with? Make a list of all the things you love doing. Now look at your list and check how many of these things you actually fill your day with. Aim to do at least three activities every day which fill you with happiness. It can be as simple as spending time with the kids, soaking in a relaxing bath or taking the dog for a walk.

Make time to meditate every day. This effectively releases emotional and mental stress.

Relax into the centre of your being. When you find yourself resting there, ask your neck what it wants you to pay attention to, such that if you were to pay attention to it the neck pain would go away?

In the coaching programme pay special attention to your values, releasing negative emotions and limiting beliefs, design your ideal day and solving difficult problems.

When to see an osteopath or chiropractor

• When injury is acute and the neck stiffens up, movement is restricted, and/or numbness, pins and needles or muscle weakness can be felt in the neck, shoulder, arm, forearm, hand or fingers
• If you have both neck pain and headaches
• If you have had neck pain for more than a few weeks
• If you have osteoarthritis in your neck
• If you have a prolapsed disc

After a whiplash injury, the earlier you seek treatment the better. But if it is very severe you must first be checked out at the hospital, although your osteopath or chiropractor will send you for further investigations if necessary.

When to see a medical doctor

• If you have pain in the neck, back of the head and difficulty swallowing, and your head is held rigidly
• Have a history of illness and low-grade fever
• Start to experience dizziness or loss of balance
• Feel like fainting when you bend your head backwards
• Have wasting of muscles in one hand, drooping of one eyelid, decreased facial sweating on one side and one pupil is contracted
• Are losing weight, have loss of appetite, or have unexplained fever, chills or night sweats
• Have hair or nail changes, feel very tired, have temperature intolerance, cramps, swelling, increased urinary frequency and unexplained weakness
• Have a cough and night sweats
• Have pain in neck, bilateral shoulders and have scalp tenderness

• Have ringing in the ears, blurred vision, light sensitivity, weakness and sweating
• Have voice changes
• Can see that your neck/throat area looks bigger than before

Which therapies help?

Osteopathy and chiropractic help by restoring optimal function of the structures that are causing the pain. It is especially useful for neuro-musculo-skeletal problems.

Acupuncture helps in both acute and chronic cases of neck pain.

Massage helps in chronic cases of neck pain and when the pain is related to stress.

Aromatherapy is particularly good when there is more of a neck tension, rather than a pain. The oils work on the whole body-mind framework and help to soothe away worries.

Healing helps especially when there is an imbalance within the emotional and mental body.

The Alexander technique, Pilates and yoga are excellent forms of exercise, which are designed to bring more awareness of the individual's posture and overall musculo-skeletal balance. In yoga and Pilates it is important to avoid those postures which increase the strain on the neck, such as headstands, shoulderstands, the Plough, the Swan Dive and the Cobra.

Hypnotherapy, NLP and well-being coaching help when you find that you allow negative emotions or stress to get to you. These therapies enable you to understand the root cause of your behaviour pattern, and help you release it and find a new, more balanced way of being.

useful affirmations

"It is safe for me to relax and trust that life is perfect just as it is."

"I can only give to others that which I have first given to myself."

"It is okay for me to take time out for myself. I am worth it."

Osteoarthritis (OA)

This is a degenerative form of arthritis, which affects the joints, especially the hips, knees, spine, wrists, feet and hands. It is the most common form of arthritis, and can be primary, often referred to as 'wear and tear', or secondary as a result of a predisposing factor, such as a previous joint fracture, hyper mobility (joints move too much, such as in some dancers and some gymnasts) or inflammatory joint disease.

Who does it affect?

Most of us will show some mild form of arthritis after the age of fifty, but it can even be present at age twenty-five, especially if there has been a previous history of fractures, or excessive physical exercise.

What are the common symptoms?

Symptoms can range from mild pain and stiffness to total loss of joint function. It is aggravated by activity and relieved by rest. Typically there is stiffness in the mornings, and the pain gradually builds up during the day as the joint is being used.

How does OA affect various joints differently?

OA of the spine often leads to pain and vascular insufficiency as the degenerated joint can start to compress on nearby nerves and blood vessels. OA of the hip leads to pain, contracture of hip flexors and decreased range of movement, whilst OA of the knee leads to pain and joint instability.

What are the psychosomatic causes?

Osteoarthritis may be indicative of someone who has difficulty moving through the changes of life. He tries to hold on to everything, causing much frustration, anger and sadness. Or he feels as if he never moved in the direction that he wanted to go in, and now feels stuck and unable to change direction. This gives rise to feelings of resentment and bitterness. For instance, someone with arthritic fingers may be feeling that everything is slipping away from him, so he tries to hold on, causing feelings of frustration and restriction. Or it may be that he feels he would like to punch someone, but instead of allowing the anger to be expressed and released, he holds it in, causing pain, tension, restriction and finally destruction of the joints. Arthritis may also be due to unexpressed frustration, such as when someone knows he is in the wrong job, but feels unable to change. This frustration has to go somewhere, and because the frustration is due to an inability to move forward in life, it symbolically starts to affect the joints, which are the parts of our body that allow for movement.

What is the most common conventional treatment of OA?

The most common conventional treatment for OA are NSAIDs (non steroidal anti-inflammatories), but although these painkillers reduce pain by stopping the pain signals reaching the brain, the pain is there for a reason—to make you do something about it. Stopping your brain from registering the pain will not help you deal with the original problem.

What are the side effects of NSAIDs?

NSAIDs increase the risk of gastro-intestinal bleeding, ulceration and perforation, especially when taken daily over a long period of time. They are very dangerous for the elderly or for those with a history of peptic ulcers. NSAIDs have also been shown to increase the destruction of cartilage, thereby aggravating the progression of osteoarthritis (41,42).

How can I help in regards to my diet?

• If the body is very toxic, a fast may be required. Only do this under supervision.
• Drink 6–8 glasses of filtered water per day to flush out toxins and avoid dehydration. Chronic pain has been associated with long-standing dehydration.
• Fresh cherries and blueberries are beneficial since they contain compounds that can decrease joint inflammation.
• Maximise intake of vegetables and fruits since they have an alkaline effect and are rich in anti-oxidants.

What should I avoid?

• Avoid dairy products, refined foods, meat, citrus fruits and margarine.
• Avoid nightshade foods (tomatoes, eggplant, white potatoes and peppers) if a sensitivity to these has been noticed, since they may aggravate the inflammatory response.
• Avoid caffeine, alcohol and tobacco.
• Avoid any known allergy foods, since these foods have been associated with osteoarthritis.
• Avoid iron supplements, since it may be involved in joint destruction due to a pro-oxidant effect.

How else can I improve my physical health?

• Maintain normal weight to avoid adding weight-bearing stress on the joints.
• Regular manipulative care is beneficial to address structural/postural problems.
• Copper bracelets may be of help.

Which supplements and herbs help?

• Calcium and magnesium are essential for bone/ligament and muscle health.
• B-complex, especially B6, vitamin A, zinc and copper help to manufacture and repair cartilage.
• Vitamin C aids in collagen formation and cartilage growth.
• Vitamin E helps to inhibit OA's progression.
• Selenium and zinc are useful.
• Cod liver oil and fish oil decrease inflammation. One study in Sweden found that 10 grams of fish oil per day had a similar anti-inflammatory effect as NSAIDs, except it did not have any of the side effects (43).
• Lactobacillus acidophilus and bromelain aid digestion.
• Glucosamine sulphate is good for enhancing cartilage production and to improve its ability to act as a shock absorber. Studies have proven it to be very effective and far superior to ibuprofen (44,45).
• Yucca and devil's claw are useful anti-inflammatory herbs.
• Shark cartilage may aid in decreasing joint inflammation and pain.
• Propolis (bee pollen) and black currant seed oil may be helpful.
• Feverfew decreases inflammation by inhibiting compounds that cause inflammation.

How can I improve my emotional, mental and spiritual health?

Daily meditation helps to balance the emotions and the mind.

Visualise yourself in perfect health. See how you move with ease through life, embracing the new, and letting go of the old.

A good meditation is to see yourself sitting at a riverbank, looking out at the River of Life. See an empty boat approach. This boat is coming to help you clear away the old. Once the boat has stopped just in front of you, tie it to the shore and put everything you no longer need in the boat. This may be old negative emotions, old beliefs, old attitudes, your job, a way of being, people, anything which is stopping you from moving forward easily and effortlessly. When you have put all that you no longer need in the boat, take the time to say everything you need to say to everyone and everything in the boat, and ask what positive lessons they have brought to you. Keep doing this until you find it in your heart to say that you love and forgive everything that is in the boat. Then say good-bye and cut the rope that ties the boat to the shore. See it float down the river, until it completely disappears in the distance. Now look out at this River of Life. State what qualities and new ways of being you now desire in your life. See the river bring you a gift, which symbolises your wishes. Take this gift inside your heart and feel its qualities fill your whole being.

With the aid of the coaching programme release all negative emotions, limiting beliefs and pain held in body tissues or caused by unwanted states and behaviours. Do the exercises for forgiveness and for solving difficult problems.

Which therapies help?

Osteopathy and cranial osteopathy help establish what has caused the increased strain on the affected joint, release the tension around the area, encourage better joint nutrition and mobility, and make sure nerve, blood and lymphatic supply are adequate to the affected and nearby structures.

Pilates helps by restoring balance within your whole body.

Healing – All forms of healing are of benefit for any type of arthritis, since they can effectively and gently release pent-up negative emotions from the body-mind framework.

Homeopathy has many remedies, which may be of help.

Kinesiology helps by assisting in restoring balance within the musculo-skeletal system. Many osteopaths, chiropractors and physiotherapists are trained in applied kinesiology.

Yoga and Pilates – If you are only suffering from mild arthritis, these forms of exercises are highly beneficial. If your joints are severely affected, both yoga and Pilates are still great, but you need to be supervised by a qualified practitioner who is also an osteopath, chiropractor or physiotherapist, since your exercises need to be modified according to your individual ability.

Hypnotherapy, NLP and well-being coaching help since arthritis often is linked with repressed negative emotions, such as anger, bitterness, frustration and fear. These forms of therapies help by releasing negative emotions, enabling you to accept life as it is, and seeing how much love and joy there is in your life already.

Useful affirmations

"It is now safe for me to move with ease through life."

"I now let go of the old and embrace the new."

"My life is filled with happiness and joy."

"You love someone truly the moment you set them free."

"Everything changes, except Love, which is eternal."

Osteoporosis

Osteoporosis is literally translated as 'porous bone'. It usually affects postmenopausal Caucasian or Asian women with a small, thin frame and a family history of osteoporosis. The entire skeleton may be involved, but usually the bone loss is greatest in the spine, hips and ribs. Since we carry a lot of weight on these bones, they are susceptible to deformity and fracture.

How common is it?

Osteoporosis in men and women accounts for over 60,000 hip, 50,000 wrist and 40,000 spinal fractures every year in the UK alone, and it affects more than 20 million people in the United States.

How is it different from osteomalacia?

Osteoporosis is very different from osteomalacia. In osteomalacia, there is only a deficiency of calcium in the bone, usually due to a lack of vitamin D, which stimulates the absorption of calcium. In osteoporosis there is a lack of both calcium and other minerals, as well as a reduction of the organic matrix (non minerals) of the bone.

What causes osteoporosis?

• Hormonal imbalance as it occurs in menopause, due to a decrease in oestrogen and progesterone levels.

• Lifestyle, such as alcohol abuse, cigarette smoking, lack of exercise or excessive exercise, intake of caffeine, carbonated drinks, refined foods, excess salt, excess fat and a high intake of protein all increase the risk of osteoporosis by increasing the loss of calcium. For example, the body always maintains equal levels of phosphorus and calcium in the blood. When you drink carbonated drinks which contain high levels of phosphorus, the body leaches calcium from the bones to maintain this equal level.

• Excess levels of phytic and oxalic acids from some cereals

• Excessive use of antibiotics. This decreases the levels of the friendly gut bacteria, which is very important for the production of vitamin K—a vital ingredient for building bone.

• Excess levels of sodium fluoride in water

• Medications such as heparin, cortico-steroids, gluco-corticoids and anti-convulsants, such as phenobarbital and phenytoin

• Anorexia or decreased body fat decreases the body's progesterone level, which is needed for the building of bone.

• Cooking with aluminum, since the parathyroid gland can be inhibited by aluminum, which can lead to osteoporosis.

• Endocrine disorders, such as thyrotoxicosis, hyperparathyroidism, Cushing's syndrome, hypergonadism, hyperadrenacorticism and diabetes mellitus.

Other causes include alcoholism, bilateral removal of ovaries, osteogenesis imperfecta, multiple myeloma, Marfan's syndrome, chronic obstructive pulmonary disease, gastrectomy, Ehler-Danlose syndrome, rheumatoid arthritis, metabolic acidosis, homocysteinuria, and immobilization. Recent research from Sweden has indicated that high levels of vitamin A may also be a factor.

What are the psychosomatic factors?

Osteoporosis may be an indication of a weakening of our support system in life. The skeleton is the support structure for the whole body, so a thinning of the bones may mean that we are lacking in social, emotional and/or mental support, either from ourselves or from our environment. It may also be a sign of severe self-doubt.

When should I contact my medical doctor?

You should contact your medical doctor immediately if you suffer from any of the following:

• If you suffer severe pain after a fall

• Start to develop a curvature of the spine

• Start decreasing in height

• Have severe backache with no apparent cause

• Have a history of any of the causes listed above

How is it commonly treated?

The most common form of orthodox treatment is oestrogen therapy which is known to slow down bone loss, but has no effect on building new bone. The risk of long-term use of these supplements is increased fat production, liver problems, increased risk of uterine and breast cancer and water retention. It has recently been stopped as a treatment.

How can my diet improve my health?

• Drink a small amount of fresh lemon juice every day, since this aids digestion.

• A vegetarian diet seems to protect against osteoporosis, possibly due to decreased bone loss in later years.

• Increase consumption of fruits and vegetables (aim for your diet to be 60–70% fruits and vegetables), especially flavonoid-rich foods (high in vitamin C), such as red and blue-black berries, colourful fruits, and calcium-rich foods, such as leafy green vegetables, fish, tofu, yoghurt, beans, fish, sesame and pumpkin seeds. The green, leafy vegetables are rich in vitamin K, which is needed to convert inactive osteocalcin to active osteocalcin and helps to anchor calcium in bone.

• Increase foods rich in boron, such as nuts, avocados, kidney and borlotti beans. Boron has been shown to increase bone health.

• Increase consumption of whole grains, nuts

and seeds, since they are an excellent source of calcium, as well as a good source of essential fatty acids.

• Increase consumption of phytoestrogen-rich foods, such as soya bean, papaya, carrots, apples, brown rice, whole wheat, sesame seeds, and fennel. Phytooestrogens have weak oestrogenic activity, and can help to increase overall oestrogen levels in the body.

• Increase intake of fish. It is especially good to eat the bones of small fish, such as sardines.

• Eat live yoghurt daily with lactobacillus bacteria to help keep a healthy gut, which is vital for the absorption of calcium.

What should I avoid?

• Avoid caffeine, alcohol and carbonated drinks, since these leach calcium out of bones.

• Avoid refined foods, sweets (sugar increases the excretion of calcium in the urine), soft drinks, fried foods, and fatty foods. The latter contain fatty acids that interfere with calcium absorption.

• Decrease intake of animal protein, except fish.

• Decrease intake of cereals, due to its excess of phytic and oxalic acids.

• Possibly decrease intake of nightshade foods (tomato, potato, eggplant and pepper) if a sensitivity to these has been noticed.

• Avoid taking vitamin A supplements.

Which supplements may be useful?

• Take a daily calcium supplement, since it has been shown to slow down the rate of osteoporosis, and may even prevent it (46,47).

• It is important that magnesium is also included, since calcium supplementation without magnesium can lead to a deficiency in magnesium and an increased risk of too much calcium in the blood, which would reduce the calcium in bones, as well as increase the risk of developing kidney stones. Magnesium has been shown

to help in the treatment of osteoporosis as well as to help prevent it (48).

• A boron supplement may be needed.

• A good B-complex is needed—especially B6, B12 and folic acid—for proper homocysteine levels. If there is a lack of these vitamins, homocysteine levels may rise, and since homocysteine can interfere with cross-linking of collagen, it can result in a weakening of the bone matrix.

• Take daily supplements of flax seed oil for the essential fatty acid content.

How else can I improve my physical health?

Make sure you get exposure to sunlight. This is essential for the synthesis of vitamin D, which is vital for the absorption of calcium and phosphorus from the intestines. If it is not possible to get enough exposure to daylight then it may be necessary to supplement with vitamin D (400 IU per day).

Weight-bearing exercise aids in building bone.

How else can I improve my emotional, mental and spiritual health?

Meditating and breathing exercises help calm the mind. Deep breathing also helps improve the function of the thoracic spine.

Enjoy just being in the here and now.

With the aid of the coaching programme release all negative emotions, limiting beliefs and do the exercise for forgiveness.

A good visualisation is to picture yourself in perfect health. See yourself standing tall and strong, and see your skeleton growing stronger and healthier. Make this internal picture very colourful and vibrant. Make sure that you see yourself clearly in the picture. Do this every day, whilst repeating affirmations to yourself, such as, "Every day, in every way, my skeleton is growing stronger and stronger."

Ease the pressure you put on yourself and on others. Make it a priority to relax and pamper yourself weekly by doing things just for you.

Learn to say 'no' when you feel you actually do not have the energy for doing something.

Remember you have all the resources you need within you. If at times you feel you are lacking in support from your environment, know that you are the only being who can give you what you truly need.

You can only give to others what you first have given to yourself.

Which therapies help?

Osteopathy and cranial osteopathy help to relieve symptoms and pain from disfigurations and previous fractures.

Yoga and Pilates help to balance the musculo-skeletal alignment with gentle, yet highly powerful exercises. Make sure your instructor is capable of giving you the appropriate advice.

Tibetan, ayurvedic and Chinese medicine help to improve the overall health of the body.

Homeopathy and medical herbalism can help.

Healing helps by balancing the emotions and restoring energy levels in the body.

NLP, hypnotherapy and well-being coaching help release limiting beliefs and enable you to find the resources you have within.

Useful Affirmations

"For every breath I take I am getting stronger and healthier."

"I have all the support I need in life within me."

"I am worthy of being strong and in full health."

Pancreatitis

This is an acute or chronic inflammation of the pancreas. The symptoms of an acute episode are usually intense pain in the abdomen that may also be felt on the left side of the chest and back (worse on lying down and relieved on leaning forward), bloating, fever, nausea, vomiting and sweating. With a chronic episode the symptoms are less intense, although still serious, such as nausea, vomiting, gas, bloating, weight loss, problems with malabsorption (fats in stools), fever, upper abdominal pain and onset of diabetes.

What are the causes?

• Excessive alcohol consumption and/or drug abuse
• Poor dietary habits, such as high intake of fatty foods, refined foods and caffeine
• Food allergies
• Problems with gallbladder (gallstones or inflammation) or liver
• Viral, bacterial or intestinal infections
• Cystic fibrosis
• Obesity
• Stress

What are the psychosomatic causes?

In a psychosomatic context the pancreas represents our ability to handle love and sweetness in our lives, as well as the opposite emotions, such as anger and fear, without causing pain to self or others. An inflammation is often a sign of repressed anger, so someone suffering from pancreatitis may feel a sense of loss of love, rejection and an inner anger, which has been turned onto the self.

How can I help in regards to the diet?

• Eat five to six small meals per day, so as not to overburden the pancreas.

• Eat a wholesome diet, rich in unrefined carbohydrates, such as brown pasta, brown rice, brown bread and vegetables.

• Eat fish and chicken sparingly. Oily fish may help to decrease an inflammatory response due to its essential fatty acid content.

• Soya products are recommended for their excellent protein, lecithin and choline content. Lecithin helps to emulsify fat and choline helps to prevent and treat neurological complications of diabetes (pancreatic problem increases the risk of diabetes).

• Certain foods have an insulin effect on the body, so eat these freely. These include artichokes, brussel sprouts, green beans, garlic, cucumber, soya products and tofu, oat products, fibre, green vegetables, wheat germ and avocado. Onions and garlic can also help to lower the blood sugar levels.

• Potassium broth is useful to help restore any lost electrolytes and minerals. Drink daily.

What should I avoid?

• During an acute stage it may be necessary to go on a liquid diet.

• Avoid all alcohol, sweets, sugar, chocolate, refined and processed foods, such as white bread, white rice, biscuits, cakes, fruits and dried fruit. They will only overburden the system further and aggravate the condition.

• Avoid all caffeine (coffee, cola, chocolate), since this stimulates a stress response in the body, exhausting the adrenal glands and in this way increases the burden on the pancreas.

• Avoid any food allergies/sensitivities.

• Avoid fatty acids from meat and dairy products, since they produce arachidonic acid, which increases the inflammatory production in the body.

Which supplements and herbs help?

• Lactobacillus acidophilus may be needed to improve the gut flora.

• Pancreatic enzymes and supplementation with B-complex and/or Brewer's yeast. The latter two will help to decrease the need for insulin, aid the action of insulin as well as improving carbohydrate metabolism.

• Vitamin C with bioflavonoids is needed by insulin for its transport, helps to stabilise blood sugar levels and is required for healthy adrenal function. Bioflavonoids increases the bioavailability of vitamin C.

• Zinc, since it is involved in insulin metabolism.

• Manganese is needed for glucose metabolism.

• Magnesium is important for control of blood glucose levels and if deficient it will increase the risk of developing cardiovascular disease.

• Coenzyme Q10 helps to promote insulin production.

• Spirulina may help to decrease the need for insulin.

• Essential fatty acids, such as flax seed oil may help to decrease the inflammatory response.

How else can I improve my physical health?

• Hot and cold flannels over the pancreas as well as mid-back to stimulate circulation and nerve flow to the pancreas and liver.

• Specific Pilates exercises, such as the spinal twist and the cat to help improve the flexibility of the spinal segments responsible for proper nerve conduction to the pancreas, liver and intestines.

• Castor oil packs over the whole abdomen; liver, pancreas, spleen, stomach and intestines. This is because pancreatitis often set up a susceptibility of developing diabetes, which can affect all these organs.

How can I improve my emotional, mental and spiritual health?

• Daily meditation, breathing exercises and relaxation are important to decrease any unnecessary stress response.
• Let go of your anger and sadness. Do the forgiveness exercise in regards to everyone you have a close relationship with. Then also do it in regards to yourself, so that you learn to forgive yourself fully.
• If needed find someone who can help you in letting go of all negative emotions, limiting beliefs and unwanted states and behaviours.
• See the love and beauty in everyone and everything. Learn to respond with love instead of anger or fear.
• Two good visualisations to do are the following:
—Sit down comfortably and go deep within in, to that still inner place. Then place your awareness in your heart. Now see a stage in front of you and place everyone you know on this stage. Take the time to tell each person on this stage what you love about them, and while you do this, keep sending them love from your heart. Keep doing this until you have spoken to all of them. Then thank them for listening and say good-bye to them.
—Now see yourself sitting on this stage. Ask all the people you know who love you to come and stand before this stage, and let each one of them tell you what they love about you, and allow your heart to open up to receive the love they are sending you. Then thank them for sharing this with you, and wish them well on their journey through life.
• Realise you are a magnificent being made of pure love. That is your pure spiritual essence, and your birth right.

Which therapies help?

Tibetan, ayurvedic or Chinese medicine and acupuncture help greatly by improving the function of the pancreas, liver and digestive tract, as well as working on the emotions.

Osteopathic and chiropractic treatment help by working to improve the function of the pancreas, kidneys, liver, gastrointestinal tract and adrenal glands by improving the nerve, blood and lymphatic flow. Various exercises may be given to improve the function of the spine.

Cranial Osteopathy uses slightly different techniques to achieve the same aim as in above, but may also be able to help to decrease the inflammatory response of the body. Some cranial osteopaths are also skilled in releasing negative emotions held within the body tissues.

Reflexology helps by stimulating the pressure points for the pancreas, liver and digestive tract.

Medical herbalism has several herbs, which are very beneficial. See a practitioner for individual advice.

Healing is very useful, especially when the emotions are unbalanced, and the energy of the body is being drained by negative emotional and mental behaviour patterns.

NLP, Hypnotherapy and Well-Being Coaching help by releasing negative emotions, aid in forgiveness and by releasing any parts conflicts within the mind, which are responsible for any addictive behaviour.

Useful affirmations

"I am worthy of love just as I am."

"The universe is filled with love everywhere. All I need to do is to be open to it."

"It is now safe for me to let go of my anger."

"As I forgive others I set myself free."

"As I forgive myself I set myself free."

Pregnancy and Associated Conditions

Pregnancy is a highly demanding time for a woman, because it requires a lot of energy to make a healthy baby. It is estimated that the energy consumption during a pregnancy is the same as running 30 marathons. This is why even a slight imbalance in the woman's well-being can have serious effects on the health of the baby and the mother.

How can I improve my baby's health?

The importance of prenatal planning

Your baby can only develop from the energy and health that is inherent within you and your partner. This is why prenatal planning is so important, and why it is good to let your body rest for 3 to 5 years between pregnancies. This allows time for the mother's body to restore her energy reserves, so that enough energy is available for the making of another healthy child. The first three months of fetal development are the most crucial, since cell division is the most prolific during this time. At twelve weeks all the organs are fully formed. It is vital to stop smoking, avoid smoky environments and avoid alcohol when you start planning for a pregnancy, since you will probably not realise you are pregnant for at least the first six weeks, and may unintentionally harm your baby.

Nutrition and pregnancy

It is important to have optimum nutrition during pregnancy, as it can greatly improve the chances of having an easy pregnancy and a healthy baby. In the past there was less pollution and the food was of a better quality; now our bodies have to fight against pesticides, exhaust gases, heavy metal toxicity, smoking and alcohol in much larger quantities than before. This is probably also one of the causes why 10–25% of all pregnancies end in miscarriage. The figure might even be higher than that, because many miscarriages go unnoticed.

Alcohol and pregnancy

In Britain it is sometimes advised that you can drink up to one unit of alcohol per day during the pregnancy. In Scandinavia it is advised that you completely abstain from alcohol throughout your pregnancy and while breastfeeding. Even small amounts of alcohol affect the absorption of nutrients in the gut, interfere with normal metabolism and can cause vital nutrients to leach out of body tissues, leading to nutritional deficiencies. During pregnancy, alcohol crosses the placenta and reaches the baby's bloodstream, causing a direct effect on the developing fetus. In breast feeding it reaches the baby through the breast milk. A mother may rationalise having a glass of wine in the evening with the reasoning that her baby will sleep better. But would you give alcohol to a toddler? Of course not. Then why to a baby? Personally, I think abstaining completely from alcohol is the safest way, but if you and your baby are otherwise healthy, an occasional small amount of a weak alcoholic drink in the later stages of pregnancy, is unlikely to cause any real damage, although it certainly will not be healthy for your baby.

Sugars and pregnancy

High levels of sugar in the diet, such as from cakes, chocolate, sugary drinks and white sugar in coffee and tea are a common cause of blood sugar swings. In pregnancy it can interfere with normal metabolism, and some research has indicated this as a contributory factor to low birth weight. It only seems to be glucose that is responsible for this (white sugar), not fructose (fruit sugar) or lactose (milk sugar).

Coffee and pregnancy

Drinking more than four cups of coffee a day is linked to an increased risk of miscarriage. It is not healthy for anyone to drink more than 1–2 cups of coffee a day. Caffeine stimulates increased adrenaline production from the adrenal glands, leading to a rise in blood glucose levels, which in turn increases the insulin production from the pancreas. It also decreases the functioning of the immune system. Remember that tea, chocolate and cola all contain high levels of caffeine.

How can I improve my baby's emotional, mental and spiritual health?

Your baby is part of your unconscious mind, so you have a very deep connection with him or her from the start. This is why many mothers-to-be know instinctively when they become pregnant, if all is well with their baby, and even what sex their baby is. Trust this connection and during your pregnancy take the opportunity to build on this bond by following the advice listed below. This will help both of you enormously.

Communicate lovingly with your baby because it picks up on your thoughts, emotions and words.

Meditate daily and send your baby as much love as you possibly can.

Visualise your baby inside your body regularly. Notice what he/she feels like, and ask if he/she needs anything from you, such as some specific foods, that you relax more or perhaps that you take the time to just have fun and laugh a lot. Perhaps he/she is perfectly content.

From time to time, visualise the labour and birth of your baby being a happy, relaxed and safe event (use goal setting). This gives direct instructions to you and your baby's unconscious minds that this is what you wish for. Ask the baby when you meditate what type of birth is prefered. Trust all the answers that come to you.

Meditate on how much love and happiness you can bring to your child, and visualise how this love and happiness creates a golden light, which shines forth into your child's future.

How can I help improve my own health in regards to my diet?

• Always have breakfast, and never skip a meal. It is better to eat frequent, small meals.
• Eat plenty of vegetables and fruits. They are an excellent source of vitamins and minerals. Try to always choose organic products.
• Eat whole grain products (bread, pasta, rice).
• Increase your consumption of pumpkin, linseed, sunflower and sesame seeds for their essential fatty acid, vitamin and mineral content.
• Try to sprinkle some wheatgerm on your food, since this is an excellent source of B-vitamins, iron and essential fatty acids.

If you have been advised not to eat dairy products, then make sure you get adequate calcium intake from seeds, pulses, vegetables and tofu. Many soya milks have added calcium.

What should I avoid?

• Avoid refined white products (bread, pasta, rice).

- Do not eat sweets, sugar, dried fruit or drink sweet drinks. Always dilute fruit juices. This is to make sure blood sugar levels remain stable.
- Do not drink alcohol, and preferably no cola, coffee or tea. If you need your cup of coffee or tea in the morning, then limit it to only one cup per day.
- Avoid fatty fish (herring, mackerel, salmon), since they are likely to have high levels of heavy metals in them (due to our polluted seas).

What about supplementation and herbs?

Supplementation is okay during pregnancy provided it is done with care. Never take extra vitamin A (avoid cod liver oil). Use a good quality multivitamin and mineral product that is specially formulated for pregnancy, and possibly a B-complex.

Take extra supplementation of organic flax seed oil; a pregnant woman's brain shrinks due to the baby depleting the mother's fatty acid stores from the brain, which is why you seem to lose your memory when pregnant.

Raspberry leaf tea during the last month of pregnancy helps to strengthen the muscles of the uterus, which helps with contractions during labour. Ask a medical herbalist for advice if your previous labour was really quick or if you have had problems with the strength of your cervix.

How else can I improve my physical health?

As soon as you start thinking about getting pregnant, start improving your whole neuro-musculo-skeletal structure through exercises, such as yoga and Pilates. The stronger and more balanced your body is, the easier it will be for you to carry the baby.

If needed, have complementary treatments, such as osteopathy and chiropractic to improve your neuro-musculo-skeletal health, and acupuncture, herbs and reflexology to improve your energy levels. This helps your body create a healthy baby.

If you have suffered from pelvic congestion, before you become pregnant, do regular sitz baths and hot and cold treatment on your lower back to improve circulation to all pelvic organs.

How can I improve my emotional, mental and spiritual health during pregnancy?

Meditate daily. This allows you to connect with your whole being—body, mind and spirit.

Take time to reflect on the coming changes. How do you feel about becoming a mother? What values do you have about motherhood? Make a list of them and see if there are any away from values in there (see values in coaching programme).

With the coaching programme release negative emotions and limiting beliefs. Do the exercises for solving difficult problems and for forgiveness (especially in regards to your own parents). When you do all this work before your child is born, you release your child from having to inherit your negative emotions and thought patterns and it frees you to be the mother you truly want to be.

Visualise yourself as the mother you wish to be. See, feel and hear yourself being all the qualities you wish to be and acting the way you wish to act. See how much happiness this brings to your child. Now take this picture and do the goal setting exercise from the coaching programme.

Know that when you are happy and balanced, everyone in your family feels truly blessed, and as they feel blessed this blessing comes back to you.

Common Ailments During Pregnancy

Anaemia

Fairly common in pregnancy due to the iron requirements by the fetus for its growth. Usually the anaemia is mild and may be due to an iron deficiency. However, it can also be due to vitamin B12, folic acid and B6 deficiency.

How can I improve my physical health?

- It is important to eat plenty of iron-rich foods, such as green leafy vegetables, wheat germ, pumpkin, sesame and sunflower seeds.
- Small amounts of organic, dark chocolate are an excellent and yummy source of iron.
- Gentle breathing exercises will help to oxygenate your blood.
- Allow yourself to rest and sleep a lot.

Which supplementation may help?

Iron supplementation may be needed at times, but unfortunately it often leads to a zinc deficiency, since iron counteracts zinc. A zinc deficiency can alter the development of the baby's immune system, and zinc deficient babies also tend to be more hyperactive and have an increased risk of developing learning difficulties. Therefore if you take extra iron in the morning, take a zinc supplement just before you go to bed. A good, gentle supplement is Floradix.

How can I improve my emotional, mental and spiritual health?

Meditate daily. Ask your anaemia what it needs you to do or pay attention to for it to improve. Trust your inner instincts.

Learn to say 'no', and start scaling down on your responsibilities. You need this time to focus on you and your baby's well-being.

A good visualisation is the following: Sit comfortably. Open up the soles of your feet and let all your tiredness drain away from your body into the ground. Feel how the earth transforms it into positive energy. Now visualise an energising red light flowing up from the ground through the soles of your feet and slowly filling your whole body. Then open up the top of your head and let universal white light energy flow down through your head filling every cell of your being. Feel the two different types of energies flowing like two currents in your body. Keep doing this until you feel thoroughly energised.

Which therapies help?

Tibetan, ayurvedic and Chinese medicine, acupuncture, cranial osteopathy, reflexology, acupressure and shiatzu all may provide help.

Constipation

A common complication of pregnancy, and it can also aggravate the tendency to develop varicose veins and haemorrhoids (see **Constipation**).

Heartburn and indigestion

A common occurrence as the baby grows (see **Common Gastro-intestinal Conditions**).

Leg, feet and toe cramps

may be due to nutrient imbalances, increased strain on the lower limbs due to altered posture and weight increase, and poor circulation to the legs and feet due to the baby compressing the arteries and veins.

How can I improve my physical health?

• Increase consumption of calcium and magnesium rich foods (see Therapies). Dairy products are not recommended because they are mucous forming. Although they are rich in calcium, they are also low in magnesium and you need both for the body to absorb calcium properly.
• Massage your legs regularly to aid circulation.
• Lie with your legs raised to aid circulation.
• Enjoy backstroke swimming.

How can I improve my emotional, mental and spiritual health?

Meditate and relax daily.

Do the same meditations as recommended in anaemia and for common female conditions.

Which therapies help?

Tibetan, ayurvedic and Chinese medicine, acupuncture, cranial osteopathy, reflexology, acupressure and shiatzu may provide help.

Morning sickness

One of the most common problems in the early stages of pregnancy, which is unfortunate, since optimum nutrition is so vital during these first weeks. In many ways it protects the baby by making sure the mother cannot stand the smell of pollutants and some foods, usually the less healthy ones. It is still important to eat, but may be easier with small, frequent meals.

How can I improve my physical health?

Before rising from bed in the morning, have a cup of ginger tea and some dried wholemeal toast. This will help to stabilise blood sugar levels.

Sleep as much as you need to. Do not be surprised if you need to go to bed at 8 pm, or if you fall asleep at the most unusual times during the day. Your body is only telling you that it needs to restore its energy reserve.

Which supplements and herbs may help?

Supplement with a vitamin B-complex and vitamin C with bioflavonoids.

Some may wish to supplement with a vitamin and mineral complex, but make sure it is formulated for pregnancy.

Ginger capsules may help with nausea.

A few drops of pure aromatherapy ginger oil on a piece of cotton wool inside your bra can help.

How can I improve my emotional, mental and spiritual health?

Meditate on your nausea. What is it trying to communicate to you? Perhaps it is your body's way of warning you of harmful foods and environments for your baby? Maybe it wants you to slow down and relax?

Know that the nausea will pass. Nearly all women feel nauseous during the first trimester, and often it is a healthy sign of a good pregnancy. So relax and trust your body.

Which therapies help?

Tibetan, ayurvedic and Chinese medicine, acupuncture, cranial osteopathy, reflexology, acupressure and shiatzu all may provide help.

Musculo-skeletal problems

such as neck pain, headaches, lower back and leg pain are fairly common during pregnancy, due to the developing fetus placing an increased strain on the mother's spine, as well as the changes occurring within the pelvis to allow for normal childbirth (see Back Pain, Neck Pain and Headaches).

Pre-eclampsia

is relatively common in pregnancy. The first signs are usually a rise in blood pressure, swelling around the ankles and protein in the urine. This can develop into eclampsia, which can be life threatening to both the mother and the baby. Since the mother usually is unaware of her illness, prenatal check-ups are vital.

What are the possible causes?

Pre-eclampsia and eclampsia have been linked to a variety of factors, one being the incomplete formation of the placenta, which can affect the immune function in the mother.

B6 deficiency has been shown in some research to be linked to these conditions as well as high copper levels. The latter may be due to a zinc deficiency, which allows the copper levels to rise.

How can I improve my physical health?

Protein deficiency can lead to oedema, and it is therefore important to have an adequate intake of protein throughout the pregnancy.

Any food allergies and/or sensitivities must also be addressed.

Calcium and magnesium supplementation as well as evening primrose oil can help to lower blood pressure and prevent pre-eclampsia.

A B-complex may be useful.

How can I improve my emotional, mental and spiritual health?

Meditate to calm your nervous system and lower your blood pressure.

Ask your pre-eclampsia what it wants you to learn or know, the learning or knowing which will help it to improve.

What is causing you tension in your life? Make a list of it, and take steps to change it.

With the help of the coaching programme release past negative emotions and do the forgiveness exercise in relation to all the key people in your life.

Which therapies help?

Tibetan, ayurvedic and Chinese medicine, acupuncture, cranial osteopathy, reflexology, acupressure and shiatzu may help as preventative measures.

Stretch marks

are common in pregnancy because of the rapid development of the fetus. They usually occur on the thighs, abdomen and breasts. They occur more often in women who have rapid weight increase, and may at times be linked to nutrient deficiencies, such as zinc, and vitamins C and E.

How can I improve my physical health?

Eat plenty of pumpkin seeds for their zinc content, fresh fruits and vegetables for their vitamin C content and seeds and wheat germ for their vitamin E content.

Moisturise with cocoa butter every day throughout the pregnancy to soften the skin.

How can I improve my emotional, mental and spiritual health?

Feel happy about your body, how it is changing and how wonderful it is for allowing this new life to come into this world.

Meditate on how your body is stretching to accommodate this new little life, and then expand this awareness to include how your emotional, mental and spiritual bodies are also expanding to accommodate and welcome this new spirit into your world.

Which therapies help?

Massage, aromatherapy massage and lymphatic drainage can help.

Haemorrhoids and varicose veins

are caused by increased intra-abdominal pressure and a restriction of blood flow from the feet and legs returning to the large vein in the groin on its way up to the heart. When this vein is compressed by the baby or by constipation, the blood flow has to take alternative routes, which means via the smaller veins (see **Haemorrhoids** and **Varicose Veins**).

Rheumatoid Arthritis (RA)

This is a chronic inflammatory condition that affects the entire body, but particularly the synovial membranes and periarticular structures (membranes lining the joints), which become swollen and stiff. Most commonly the joints of the hands, feet, wrists, ankles and knees are involved. Usually the joints are affected symmetrically, i.e. in both hands, feet or ankles, which is in contrast to osteoarthritis where there usually is an asymmetrical involvement. However, RA can affect the joints unilaterally.

What are the symptoms?

Since RA is an autoimmune disease, where the body attacks itself, constitutional symptoms are usually present, such as low-grade fever and fatigue. Other symptoms include painful, swollen, tender joints and a purplish colour of the over-lying skin. In more advanced cases, joint deformity with contracture occurs in the hands and feet. Because it can affect any part of the body it can also involve the heart, lungs and eyes. It can give ligamentous laxity (loose ligaments) of which the upper neck joints are of most concern due to the risk of subluxation (partial dislocation), which can lead to instabitity of this important area. Even though RA is a chronic disease, it has periods where the symptoms are more or less intense, or where it seems to be in remission.

Whom does it affect?

Females are three times more likely to be affected than men and the onset usually occurs between 20–50 years of age, although it can strike at any time.

What are the causes?

The causes of RA are not fully understood, but there seem to be some contributing factors, such as genetics, abnormal bowel function, food allergies, nutritional factors, infectious agents and stress.

What are the psychosomatic causes?

RA may be an indication of an individual who is attacking herself with her own thoughts, just as RA is a disease where the body attacks itself. It may be that the individual has bottled up feelings of anger, resentment, bitterness, guilt, shame and low self-esteem for such a long time that eventually these feelings start attacking the self, when they are not being let out from the body. Perhaps the affected individual is having problems dealing with these negative emotions and setting boundaries; thereby becoming self-sacrificing, which may lead to deep criticism of self and others. This results in pain, restriction and lack of freedom.

How can I help in regards to the diet?

Societies who eat a 'primitive' diet have less incidence of RA than in the western world, so aim for your diet to be as natural as possible, rich in whole foods, brown rice and pasta, vegetables, fruits and fibre.

Aim for your diet to be 70–80% alkaline (most fruits, vegetables, millet, pulses, sprouted seeds, almonds, Brazil nuts, tofu, egg-white) and 20–30% acid (wheat, rye, barley, oat, peanuts, walnuts, lentils, cranberries, plums, prunes, meat, fish, egg yolk, sugar, honey, olives). Neutral foods are seeds, yoghurt, butter and tea.

Increase intake of green vegetables, lettuce, cabbage, brussel sprouts, broccoli, garlic, onions, apples, raisins, prunes, dates and pumpkin seeds. These are rich in essential vitamins and minerals needed for the healing of RA (especially vitamin C, manganese, zinc and sulphur).

Eat deep red and blue berries daily, such as cherries, blueberries, bilberries and hawthorn berries. They are very rich in proanthocyanidins (flavonoids), which aid in stabilising collagen and membranes.

Increase intake of fatty fish oil (herring, mackerel, salmon and sardines), since their fatty acid decreases an inflammatory response.

Eat organic as much as possible.

Drink soya milk or rice milk instead of cow's milk.

Drink 6–8 glasses of filtered or bottled water every day to help the body flush out toxins.

May need to undertake a detox of the body, which should only be done under supervision.

What should I avoid?

• Avoid smoking, alcohol, caffeine (coffee, cola, chocolate) and tea.
• Avoid refined carbohydrates, such as white rice, white pasta or white bread.
• Avoid vinegar (high in acids) and dry roasted nuts.
• Avoid any known food allergies/sensitivities. Try an elimination diet under the supervision of a qualified practitioner. Many foods can aggravate RA, but the most common ones are dairy products, red meat, citrus, wheat, corn and nightshade foods (tomatoes, eggplant, potatoes, peppers and tobacco).
• Avoid pesticides, food additives and colourings.
• Avoid fatty acids from meat and dairy products, since they produce arachidonic acid, which increases the inflammatory production in the body.

Which supplements and herbs help?

• Cod liver oil, garlic capsules, vitamin C with bioflavonoids, vitamin E and selenium aid in decreasing inflammation.
• A B-complex may be needed as well, since some B-vitamins (B3 and B5) have been reported to be low in RA patients, and supplementation seems to improve the symptoms.
• Zinc supplements may be useful, because it is often decreased in RA sufferers. (Never take it with iron, because it isn't absorbed. Instead take it on its own).
• Avoid iron supplementation, since it may have an involvement in joint destruction. Instead increase consumption of iron rich foods, such as broccoli, raisins and green, leafy vegetables.
• Lactobacillus acidophilus and bifidus (dairy free) help maintain healthy gut flora.
• Bromelain may be good as a digestive aid.
• Devil's claw, yucca, feverfew, ginger, curcumin and liquorice are very useful for their anti-inflammatory action. Ginseng may also be of help. Liquorice is good if patient is also taking NSAIDs, as it can help to protect against stomach ulcers. See a herbalist for advice.

How else can I improve my physical health?

• Castor oil packs to the liver and Epsom salt baths are useful in detoxifying the body.
• Hot and cold showers are good for stimulating the circulation (see **Therapies**).
• Copper bracelets may be of help.

How can I improve my emotional, mental and spiritual health?

Daily breathing exercise and meditation is vital. Your body and emotions are under strain from the illness, so balancing your mind and emotions daily is of utmost importance.

Learn to delegate tasks that you do not need to do. This conserves your energy, which your body can use for healing.

Learn to set boundaries and say 'no'.

Look for the positive in any situation in life.

Look at how much you already have in your life, and how in so many ways you help to improve the lives of others. Isn't it about time you learn to love and approve of yourself more?

Visualise yourself in perfect health and send your RA as much love as you possibly can. Keep sending it love until it feels complete. Then ask it what it needs from you in order for it to get better. Act on this guidance.

Another good visualisation is to imagine you are standing in front of a mirror. See your own reflection in this mirror. Just notice what you see, as you look at yourself through your own eyes. Then turn around so that you cannot see the mirror anymore. Ask all the people who truly love you to come and stand in front of you. Imagine that you float inside each of them. Go inside their hearts and feel what they feel for you and look at yourself through their eyes. Notice what they see when they look at you. Hear what they have to say to you about how much they love you, and what they appreciate the most about you. Do this for each and every one of them, and feel how good it feels. Then turn around and look at yourself in the mirror again, and this time see yourself the way they see you. Notice how much the reflection has changed. Keep this good feeling inside of you as you open your eyes.

With the coaching programme release all negative emotions, limiting beliefs and pain held in the body and do the exercises for forgiveness and solving difficult problems.

What are the orthodox treatments?

Orthodox treatment of RA has a poor track record, and the side effects of the drugs can be severe. One study that followed 112 patients over a period of 22 years, who all received aggressive orthodox treatment, showed that 54% of the patients died or became severely disabled (most of it as a direct effect of the RA). Only 18% were able to live normal lives (49). The orthodox treatment usually starts with non-steroidal anti-inflammatories (NSAIDs), then steroidal anti-inflammatories and finally rheumatic drugs, such as gold, anti-malaria drugs and cytoxic drugs. None of the NSAIDs have been shown to have better results than aspirin, but they have more severe side effects, such as increased risk of gastrointestinal bleeding, ulceration and perforation. NSAIDs are dangerous in the elderly or in those with a history of peptic ulcers. Side effects of gold and cytotoxic drugs are nausea, mouth ulcers, anorexia and bone marrow suppression.

Which therapies help?

Tibetan, ayurvedic and Chinese medicine help to restore as much health as is possible.

Cranial osteopathy helps to minimise stresses to joints due to poor posture and destruction.

Kinesiology helps to establish any food sensitivities.

Homeopathy has many remedies which help, such as bryonia (stiffness, inflammation and throbbing pain) and calcarea carbonica (for aching joints with node formation).

Medical herbalism has many useful herbs.

Healing helps to balance the emotions.

NLP, hypnotherapy and well-being coaching help release negative emotions and beliefs.

Useful affirmations

"I am worthy of love. I love and respect myself."

"It is now safe for me to let my feelings out."

"I am now able to set boundaries with love."

Thyroid Problems

The thyroid gland regulates many bodily functions, such as body temperature, metabolic rate and energy consumption, and in children it controls growth rate. The thyroid produces two hormones (T3 and T4), which are controlled by a hormone produced by the pituitary (thyroid stimulating hormone—TSH). Since thyroid hormones regulate metabolism of all body cells, a change in their secretions can affect all body functions. In hypothyroidism the thyroid gland becomes underactive and in hyperthyroidism it becomes overactive.

Hypothyroidism

When it occurs in children it leads to retarded physical and mental development.

What causes it?

95% of cases of hypothyroidism are due to primary hypothyroidism, which is due to a defective thyroid. 5% are due to secondary hypothyroidism, where the cause lies somewhere else, such as an under functioning pituitary gland leading to low TSH levels. A common cause of hypothyroidism is Hashimoto's disease, which is an autoimmune disease where the production of T3 and T4 is prevented by antibodies that have bound to the thyroid gland.

Other causes to decreased thyroid function:
• Iodine deficiency

- Other nutrient deficiencies
- Depressed immune system
- Candida
- Dysfunctions of the liver
- Disorders of the anterior pituitary
- Post-hyperthyroid surgery
- Diet pills
- Birth control pills containing oestrogen (reduces T3 uptake)
- Spinal lesions, especially C3 to T1–T2
- Certain drugs, such as lithium
- Hormonal imbalances
- Emotions. This cause is quite common because the thyroid is controlled by the pituitary and hypothalamus in the brain. Strong emotions have a direct effect on the hypothalamus, which will change its hormone production accordingly. Studies have shown that the thyroid appears to be especially vulnerable to emotional upsets, such as a divorce or bereavement (50).

What are the clinical signs?

Clinical hypothyroidism shows low levels of thyroid hormone. However, mild hypothyroidism may not show up on blood test, although the symptoms may already be there and a large number of cases may go undetected. Therefore, it is important to look for any other signs and symptoms and not only rely on blood tests.

How can I test myself for hypothyroidism?

By checking your basal body temperature. Take the body temperature at the same time for three consecutive mornings. Menstruating women need to do this on the second, third and fourth day of menstruation, post-menopausal women and men can do it at any time in the month. The body temperature should be within 97.6 and 98.2 degrees Fahrenheit. If lower than that it may be indicative of mild hypothyroidism.

What are the other signs and symptoms?

- Slow reflexes
- Fatigue, depression and weakness (usually first symptoms)
- Unexplained weight gain
- Sensitivity to cold and cold hands and feet
- Carpal tunnel syndrome (pins and needles and/or numbness in medial three fingers)
- Difficulty concentrating and memory loss
- Low body temperature (axillary below 97.5 F or 36.4 C)
- Loss of libido
- Slow speech
- Constipation
- Slow heart rate
- Hair loss
- Personality changes
- Headaches
- Recurrent or chronic infections
- Skin problems (acne, eczema, psoriasis)
- Anaemia

Symptoms are worse in the morning due to slower metabolic rate, whilst improving with exercise due to increased metabolic rate.

What are the psychosomatic causes?

In a psychosomatic context hypothyroidism may indicate a person who has lost their inner desire to live or their belief that they can fulfill their dream in life, so they lose their inner drive to create the life they want. It may reflect a person who has given up, or who is slowly allowing life to fade away, thinking 'what's the point?'

Hyperthyroidism

What are the causes?

• Nutritional deficiencies (especially A, E, B-vitamins, iodine and tyrosine)
• Tumour of the pituitary leading to an increase in TSH
• Dysfunction of liver leading to a decreased amount of enzymes needed to deactivate thyroid hormone
• Low immune system
• Increased intake of iodised salt may increase the risk, especially in women (51,52)
• Specific spinal dysfunctions leading to a change in nerve, blood and lymphatic flow to the thyroid gland
• Stress and emotions, since the hypothalamus plays an important role in the function of the thyroid gland. It is very easily affected by strong emotions and will change its hormone production accordingly.

What are the signs and symptoms?

• Weight loss despite an increased appetite
• Intolerance to heat
• Insomnia
• Restlessness, nervousness and anxiety
• Trembling
• Increased sweating
• Faster heart rate and often hypertension
• Increased body temperature (above 98.2 F)
• Diarrhoea
• Bulging, staring eyes
• The thyroid is often enlarged and nodular, so throat looks bigger.

What are the orthodox treatments?

Treatment is often through drugs or operation, but a third of all cases often improve by themselves (53). One method of drug treatment is swallowing a capsule of radioactive iodine, which will help to destroy parts of the thyroid gland. This may sometime lead to an underactive thyroid or if the patient is pregnant, the fetus may become mentally retarded and/or suffer from hypothyroidism. Another form of drug treatment is an anti-thyroid drug, such as carbimazole, methimazole or propylthiouracil, which may help the patient to achieve normal thyroid function. However, methimazole, which is the most potent one, has side-effects such as decreasing white blood cells, reducing the ability of bone marrow to make red blood cells, reducing blood platelets, and making the liver toxic. Some choose to have the operation which involves removing parts of the thyroid gland. They often have to be on medication with thyroxine for life.

What are the psychosomatic causes?

In a psychosomatic context hyperthyroidism may be an indication of a person who is very stressed, always doing things, but not doing enough of what would fulfill the self. The person may feel as if all her efforts are wasted, as if there is a black hole inside that she is trying to fill by being constantly active. The thyroid regulates vital life-sustaining processes, and it needs to have clear direction from our inner being that we do want to live.

Advice for both conditions

What can I do to help in regards to my diet?

It is very important to eat a healthy diet.

Special advice for hypothyroidism:

• Eat foods rich in iodine, such as fish, seafood, seaweed, kelp, potatoes and vegetables.

• Other foods that help to promote the function of the thyroid are garlic, egg yolks, mushrooms, wheat germ and brewer's yeast.

• Eat raw foods as much as possible, or just lightly steamed vegetables, since this allows the food to have a high bioavailability of vitamins and minerals.

• Use iodised salt sparingly. If used too much it can inhibit the synthesis of iodine.

• Avoid foods that stop the body from utilising iodine (termed goitrogens), such as turnips, mustard, cabbage, soybean, millet, broccoli, spinach, brussel sprouts, pears, peaches, pine nuts and peanuts. Once cooked these goitrogens seem to be inactivated.

Special advice for hyperthyroidism:
Increase consumption of foods that slow down the function of the thyroid gland (termed goitrogens), such as turnips, mustard, cabbage, soybean, millet, broccoli, spinach, brussel sprouts, pears, peaches, pine nuts and peanuts. Eat them uncooked as much as possible, since cooking deactivates them.

What should I avoid for both conditions?

• Avoid unhealthy foods, such as refined carbohydrates and processed foods.

• Eliminate totally coffee, tea, chocolate, nicotine, soft drinks and sugar.

Which supplements may be of benefit?

• Supplement with vitamin C, E, B-complex, beta-carotene, zinc and manganese, since they are needed for a healthy thyroid gland.

• Cod liver oil and flax seed oil may be useful, since essential fatty acids are needed for thyroid function.

Special advice for hypothyroidism:
If you are taking thyroid medication also take extra calcium and magnesium, since these medications speed up bone loss.

May be useful to take magnesium and calcium anyway, since a deficiency in thyroid hormone can lead to a deficiency in calcium.

Seaweed extract may help.

Special advice for hyperthyroidism:
Take a good multivitamin and mineral tablet so that the body will not be worn down by the increased metabolic rate. Some amino acid support may also be needed.

How else can I improve my physical health?

Hot and cold packs (see **Therapies**) over the thyroid will help to normalise its function.

Yoga postures (the Shoulder Stand and the Plough) and Pilates exercises (the Pelvic Bridge and Spinal Twist) are beneficial for healthy thyroid function.

For hypothyroidism, make sure you exercise vigourously daily, so at least a sweat breaks out, as this stimulates thyroid function and make tissues more sensitive to thyroid hormone.

How can I improve my emotional, mental and spiritual health?

Daily meditation and breathing exercises are vital to balance the body and the mind.

With the coaching programme do the exercises for negative emotions, limiting beliefs, emotional pain held in the body, forgiveness and solving difficult problems.

What is it that you truly want to do? What are your innermost dreams and desires? How would your ideal day, week and life be? Really think about these questions and set up goals for yourself to reach your dreams.

What is it that your soul has a longing to express in this life? What qualities and gifts within you would you like to share with the world? We all have unique talents that we are meant to bring forth into this life; it allows us to express our authentic self. Look deep within yourself until you find these answers. This allows you to uncover the hidden diamond within you.

Look at your life. How much of your time to you spend doing things you love doing? If it is less than 90% then look at how you can change that. Perhaps you need to change the way you work, or get someone to help you with certain tasks you do not enjoy.

Which therapies help?

Tibetan, ayurvedic and Chinese medicine and acupuncture help by normalising the function of the thyroid and the whole endocrine system.

Osteopathy, cranial osteopathy and chiropractic help by normalising the function of the thyroid gland through spinal manipulations (C3-T1/2), releasing restrictions in the upper ribcage, sterno-clavicular joints and fascia around the thyroid.

Reflexology helps by stimulating pressure points related to the thyroid.

Healing helps to balance the emotions.

NLP, hypnotherapy and well-being coaching help by releasing negative emotions and limiting beliefs and by enabling you to discover what you want to do in life.

Useful affirmations

"It is now safe for me to express myself."

"Now is the time to follow my dreams."

"As I still my mind I find the answers within."

"For every in-breath I breathe in peace and calm, and for every out-breath I release all that I do not need." (hyperthyroidism)

"For every in-breath I breathe in energy and vitality, and for every out-breath I release all that I do not need." (hypothyroidism)

Tinnitus

Tinnitus is a condition giving rise to ringing in the ears, sometimes accompanied by ear pain and occasionally dizziness.

What causes it?

The ringing sound is most often due to a nerve irritation or an underlying ear problem. Rarely is it due to an enlarged vein (hearing the blood rushing through it) which needs orthodox medical treatment.

Common causes are:
• Previous trauma to the head and/or ears
• Exposure to loud noise
• Blocked eustachian tubes
• Excess secretion of earwax
• Repeated episodes of ear infections
• Decreased circulation in the ears
• Dysfunction of the occipital – first cervical joint (where the neck meets the skull)
• Temporo-mandibular joint dysfunction
• Meniere's disease
• Tumour
• Hypertension and atherosclerosis
• Anaemia and hypoglycaemia
• High fat and cholesterol diet may decrease the amount of oxygen reaching the inner ear and therefore trigger tinnitus
• Smoking

• Hypersensitivity to salicylates (found in food and in certain drugs, such as aspirin)

What are the psychosomatic causes?

Tinnitus may be an indication that we are refusing to listen to the inner voice, the inner guidance and wisdom. When this inner voice is not being heard it will literally start ringing a warning bell in the hope that this finally will get our attention. It can also be a way of refusing to listen to something or someone from the outside environment (such as someone who is always nagging us).

How can I help in regards to the diet?

To prevent a child from developing tinnitus, breastfeed for at least six months, and avoid weaning too early. (The digestive tract is not ready to receive food until the baby is 6 months). If you follow theses guidelines the baby's immune system will function better and therefore it will be more able to fight ear infections.

Have a diet rich in fibre, essential fatty acids, vitamins and minerals, so increase consumption of fruits, vegetables, seeds and brown rice.

What should I avoid?

• Do not drink coffee, tea or alcohol
• Avoid saturated fat and cholesterol
• Avoid antibiotics when an ear infection is present, unless there is a risk of the infection spreading to the mastoid bone or the meningeal sheaths. If antibiotics are needed supplement with lactobacillus acidophilus.
• Avoid public swimming pools, loud noises and smoky environments

Which supplementation and herbs help?

• Vitamin C with bioflavonoids, beta-carotene, zinc, echinacea, goldenseal and propolis help to improve the immune system.
• Ginkgo biloba and vitamin E aid circulation.
• Garlic helps to improve the immune system and hinder atherosclerosis from building up.
• B 12 and manganese have been found to be deficient in many sufferers of tinnitus.
• Lactobacillus acidophilus improves gut flora.

How else can I improve my physical health?

• Mullein eardrops may be useful, especially if there has been a history of ear infections.
• In chronic cases, hot and cold treatment may be helpful in aiding circulation (see Therapies).

How can I improve my emotional, mental and spiritual health?

Meditate daily, since this effectively stills your mind. This allows you to start listening to your inner voice and helps you to remain calm and balanced when you have to deal with negative outside circumstances.

What is it your tinnitus wants you to pay attention to, know or learn, so that if you were to do that, your tinnitus would disappear?

With the aid of the coaching programme release negative emotions, emotional pain held in the body, limiting beliefs and do the forgiveness exercise.

Realise that it is perfectly safe for you to hear everything that happens in your life, because you always have the choice of whether you want to accept someone else's negativity into your own reality or not. Remember it is their stuff, not yours. It only becomes yours when you allow it to.

Which therapies help?

Osteopathy, cranial osteopathy and chiropractic help especially when the underlying cause of the complaint is of a neuro-musculo-skeletal origin, such as upper neck joint, jaw (temporo-mandibular-joint) and cranial bones (usually sphenoid, parietals, temporals and cranial base) dysfunction. This would effectively be treated and balanced.

Tibetan, ayurvedic and Chinese medicine and acupuncture help by treating the neurological, vascular and musculo-skeletal system.

Homeopathic remedies, such as calcarea carbonica (when experienced on it's own or accompanied by vertigo), cimicifuga (when accompanied with neck and back tension and sensitivity to noise) and graphites (when accompanied with deafness).

Medical herbalism has many herbs, which are suitable.

Kinesiology helps by establishing if a food sensitivity is present and also by balancing the musculo-skeletal system.

Healing helps especially when the underlying cause is of an emotional nature.

NLP, hypnotherapy and well-being coaching help by establishing the psychosomatic cause to why the ringing started in the first place, and then help you to release these emotional and mental blockages, which enables you to set up better coping strategies for the future.

Useful affirmations

"It is now safe for me to hear everything that happens in my life. When I hear something negative it is my choice if I accept that into my reality, or not."

"I am now listening to the wisdom of my inner voice."

Urinary Tract Infections

These can include an inflammation of the bladder (cystitis) and/or urethra and the kidneys (pyelonephritis). The latter is a very serious condition, which requires immediate hospitalisation.

What are the symptoms?

Cystitis gives pain and burning on urination, a need to pass urine again even after emptying the bladder, increased frequency of urination, especially at night and the urine may have a strong odor, be cloudy and dark. A slight fever may be present as well as pain in the lower abdomen.

Pyelonephritis presents with a high fever, chills, lower back pain, increased frequency of urination, pain, burning and possible blood on urination, nausea and sometimes vomiting.

What are the causes?

Urinary tract infections are caused by bacteria entering the urethra and traveling to the bladder (at times all the way to the kidneys). It is more common in females than in males, except in infants.

What makes the host more susceptible?

• It is more common in females, because the female urethra is shorter and closer to the anus, predisposing it to infection from the faeces.
• In males it may be due to an anatomical abnormality, rectal intercourse or prostate infection.
• Improper toilet habits in young girls. After emptying the bowels the genitals should be wiped separately. Clean the area around the anus from the back, wiping towards the back.

Then clean the area of the vagina from the front, wiping towards the front. In this way bacteria from the faeces cannot enter the vagina.

• Poor hygiene of genitals
• 'Honeymoon' cystitis. Frequent intercourse irritates local structures.
• Inadequate emptying of bladder, or holding on to urine for too long
• Lack of fluid, since the kidneys and urethra need fluid to flush out the build up of bacteria in the urine
• Food allergies
• Heavy metal toxicity, chemicals, drugs, birth control pills and antibiotic use
Prostate enlargement, which may block urethra
• Pregnancy
• After childbirth, the baby is not pressing on the bladder anymore and the mother does not feel when the bladder is full and so may not empty it when she ought to. It may also be due to the bladder altering its position in such a way that it retains urine.
• Constipation, which causes toxins that should have been eliminated, to be reabsorbed by the bloodstream and then handled by the kidneys.
• Poor liver function increases pressure on the kidneys
• Poor kidney function
• Spinal dysfunctions, since this may impair the proper nerve functioning of the urinary tract.
• Stress and emotions, such as anxiety and anger

What are the psychosomatic causes?

A urinary tract infection may be an indication of bottled up negative emotions, which are starting to cause us pain and anger, and we are unable to let go of them. We may not know how to express the negative feelings we feel for someone close to us, or how to deal with the situation appropriately.

How can I help in regards to the diet?

• Drink 6–8 glasses per day of filtered water.
• Drink at least 4 glasses of cranberry juice per day. Make sure it is not the drink, which contains sugar, and is not beneficial. If you cannot find pure juice, many health shops sell cranberry juice tablets. Cranberries reduce the adherence of bacteria to the lining of the urethra and bladder, and help to acidify the urine, which makes it difficult for bacteria to grow. Hippuric acid (a component of cranberry) has a slight anti-bacterial action.
• Fresh blueberries have also been found to reduce the adherence of bacteria to the walls of the bladder and urethra.
• Eat plenty of alkalising foods, such as most fruits, vegetables, millet, pulses, sprouted seeds, almonds, Brazil nuts and tofu.
• It may be useful to fast. Only undertake to do this under supervision of a qualified practitioner.

What should I avoid?

• Do not drink coffee, tea or alcohol.
• Do not eat refined foods, sugar and yeast products—the latter especially if you also suspect candida.

How else can I improve my physical health?

Once the condition has improved, alternate hot and cold sitz baths (see **Therapies**) to increase the circulation and aid the function of the urinary tract.

Yoga and Pilates exercises help improve spinal mobility and strength, as well as enhancing the tone of the pelvic floor.

Which supplements and herbs help?

• Vitamin C with bioflavonoids, vitamin A, echinacea, goldenseal and zinc are important for the immune system. Goldenseal also has anti-microbial properties and vitamin A and zinc are good for tissue healing.
• Lactobacillus acidophilus is recommended to restore gut flora. This is especially important if there is a history of antibiotic use. Take daily capsules orally and place one to two capsules in the vagina before going to bed at night every other night for a couple of weeks.
• The herb uva ursi (from upland cranberry or bearberry) has diuretic properties, and has a urinary antiseptic component (arbutin). It helps to prevent recurrent urinary tract infections.
• Garlic is useful in helping the immune system and as it also has anti-fungal properties it may help to prevent a candida infection.
• Juniper berries, celery and watermelon are good since they have diuretic qualities.

How can I prevent urinary tract infections?

• Regularly drink unsweetened cranberry juice and eat fresh blueberries. Supplement with cranberry juice tablets and uva ursi.
• Improve your immune system (see **Immune System**).
• Always clean genitals properly.
• Empty bladder and wash after intercourse.
• Always empty bladder when you feel the need to do so. If you recently have had a child remember to empty bladder regularly even if you do not feel the need to go.
• Avoid tight fitting or synthetic fibre underwear.
• Avoid bubble baths, vaginal deodorants and perfumed soaps. Use only natural soaps and essential oils (see an aromatherapist for advice).
• If any of the psychosomatic causes were true for you, then do something about it.

How can I improve my emotional, mental and spiritual health?

Practice meditation and breathing exercises daily to release negative emotions and thoughts.

Check your values for relationships, family and if needed, for work/career (see chapter on values). Are they aligned or do you detect any limiting beliefs and negative emotions there?

With the coaching programme release all negative emotions, limiting beliefs and emotional pain held in the body or caused by unwanted behaviour. Do the exercises for solving difficult emotions and for forgiveness—do it for all the important relationships in your life.

Are you able to set your boundaries with love? Or do you wait to assert yourself until you are so angry and resentful that your boundaries come storming out in a temper? Practice being firm, whilst still being calm and balanced.

Are you holding any grudges towards your partner? Write them all down. Then write down all the good things your partner does. Now pretend you are floating inside your partner, and see the situation through your partner's eyes. What different insights does this give you? From this place of expanded awareness, see what it is you need to communicate with your partner, so that you can connect with your own inner love again.

Remember that only you are responsible for your inner happiness so regularly do things that bring you pleasure and joy.

You only need love and approval from yourself, so do what you feel is right for you.

Which therapies help?

Medical herbalism is excellent in the treatment of urinary tract infections.

Tibetan, ayurvedic and Chinese medicine and acupuncture help greatly to improve the function and the health of the whole urinary tract, as well as helping to balance the emotions.

Acupressure, shiatzu and reflexology help heal through stimulating pressure points related to the urinary tract, spine, immune system, adrenal glands and digestive system.

Osteopathy and chiropractic help by restoring proper nerve, blood and lymphatic flow to the urinary tract, the immune system and gastrointestinal tract. Cranial and visceral osteopathy help to also reduce tissue tension.

Homeopathic remedies, such as berberis vulgaris (for cystitis with a burning feeling), clematis (when the person has to urinate often, with only a few drops being passed) and nux vomica (irritable bladder with frequent needs to urinate) can be helpful.

Healing helps to balance the emotions and restore lost energy within the body.

NLP, hypnotherapy and well-being coaching help especially when there are problems within personal relationships, letting go of negative emotions, or difficulty with setting boundaries safely and constructively.

Useful affirmations

"As I release the old I embrace the new into my life with love."

"It is now safe for me to state my needs and set my boundaries."

"I love and accept myself."

Varicose Veins

The veins are responsible for bringing deoxygenated blood from all the tissues in the body back to the heart where it then goes to the lungs to become oxygenated again. All veins contain valves, which prevent blood from flowing backward due to gravity. When the walls of the vein becomes weak, the vein dilates and the valve gets damaged. This leads to pooling of blood, which causes the vein to bulge, leading to varicose veins.

Who does it affect?

It affects nearly half of the middle-aged population, and women are affected four times more than men.

What are the common symptoms?

• Distended superficial veins in the legs
• It may be asymptomatic, or it may present with feelings of an aching pain and/or heaviness in the legs.
• The overlying skin may become discoloured and ulcerated.
• There may be signs of fluid retention.
• Haemorrhoids are also a type of varicose vein.

What causes it?

• The large vein in the groin can be compressed during pregnancy by the baby or by constipation; the blood flow then has to take alternative routes, which means via the smaller veins.
• Heavy lifting, vomiting, excessive coughing or straining on the toilet increases the intra-abdominal pressure, which aggravates the tendency to dilate and distend the small veins.
• Long periods of standing restrict the blood flow from the feet and legs.
• Genetic weakness of the vein walls or the valves
• Inflammation of the veins can damage the veins and/or the valves.

What are the psychosomatic causes?

Blood is a symbol for the love that circulates in our bodies and in our lives. Oxygenated blood carries the love we share with others, and the veins bring the love coming to us from the outside world back to our heart. Therefore an individual with varicose veins may be very good at giving love to others, but unable to give it to the self and/or to receive love from others. It may also be an indication that the environment we are in, or the direction we are heading in, is not nourishing us emotionally, which leaves us weakened and unsupported.

How can I help in regards to the diet?

• Drink plenty of filtered water to soften the stools and flush out toxins.
• Take a few tablespoons of whole linseeds daily to aid bowel motion.
• Take at least one tablespoon of olive oil daily to soften the stools.
• To strengthen the tissues of the veins proanthocyanidin and anthocyanidin-rich foods are very beneficial. Therefore eat lots of blue and red berries, such as strawberries, blueberries and cherries.
• Eat plenty of natural dietary fibre, such as fruits, vegetables, whole grains and legumes, so as to improve bowel function (see Constipation).

What should I avoid?

• Avoid eating a low fibre diet and refined foods.
• Do not strain when sitting on the toilet, since this increases the intra-abdominal pressure.
• Avoid standing or sitting for prolonged periods of time.
• Avoid heavy lifting.

How else can I improve my physical health?

• Exercise daily, such as walking.
• Hot and cold sitz baths are useful for increasing the circulation and therefore aiding the recovery of the affected tissues.
• Locally applied cold packs are good during acute phases, especially when there is inflammation.
• Witch hazel cream applied locally is beneficial in most cases. Also useful is a lemon juice compress.
• Pilates exercises focusing mostly on strengthening the pelvic floor, aiding the function of the diaphragm, improving spinal mobility for the segments responsible for healthy nerve flow to the digestive tract (top of neck, mid back and sacrum) and re-aligning the balance between the pelvis and lower back.
• Yoga, especially inverted postures, because they aid the venous supply, so it takes the effort out of the veins and gives them a rest.
• Rest with your legs elevated. This helps the veins bring the blood back to your heart without much effort.

Which supplements and herbs help?

• Vitamin C with bioflavonoids
• B-complex and zinc
• Vitamin A. Do not take if pregnant or if suffering from osteoporosis.
• Vitamin E aids circulation. Do not take if on warfarin.
• Horse chestnut is estimated to be as effective as compression stockings.
• Gotu kola appears to enhance connective tissue structure and improve blood flow.
• Flavonoid-rich extracts, such as pine bark and grape seed

How can I improve my emotional, mental and spiritual health?

• Learn to love yourself and to prioritise your own needs. You can only give to others that which you have first given to yourself.

• Practice saying 'no' with love, and honour your own boundaries.

• Find out your inner wishes and needs. What is important to you in life? What qualities and experiences do you need to be happy and fulfilled? Write them down, and then look for ways to incorporate this into your reality.

• If you could be, do and have anything, what would you want to do with your life? Which direction would you want to go in? What's stopping you from achieving this? Write the answers down to these questions, because it will reveal to you your inner dreams, as well as the limiting beliefs and decisions, which are blocking you from fulfilling those dreams.

• With the coaching programme release all negative emotions, limiting beliefs and do the exercise for forgiveness. This is especially important if you have a history of being abused emotionally and/or physically.

• When you release the negative emotions and limiting beliefs and allow yourself to heal fully, you free yourself from the past, and are able to live in the now as a happy and free individual.

• Daily meditation and breathing exercises strengthen your connection with your inner wisdom, calm your mind and balance your emotions.

• A good meditation to do is the following: Go within and find your inner stillness. Then place your awareness in your heart, and connect with the love that is there. Feel this love circulate all around your body until your whole body is vibrating with the energy of love. Then send this love out to everyone you know, and feel how this love is being returned to you multiplied. Allow yourself to receive this love and then send it to every cell of your being.

Which therapies help?

Tibetan, ayurvedic and Chinese medicine and acupuncture are great for improving the function of the blood circulation and the digestive system.

Osteopathy, cranial osteopathy and chiropractic help by improving the whole neuro-musculo-skeletal alignment, thereby aiding the circulatory and the digestive systems.

Pilates and yoga help to balance the whole neuro-musculo-skeletal system, which improves circulation and tissue health to all veins.

Reflexology, shiatzu and acupressure help by stimulating the energy reflexes in the body, which are related to the function of the veins.

Medical herbalism has several herbs which are useful in improving the structure and the function of the veins.

Homeopathy has many remedies that are suitable. See a homeopath for specific advice.

Healing aids in balancing the emotions as well as improving the life force within the venous tissues.

Hypnotherapy, NLP and well-being coaching help in releasing negative emotions and limiting beliefs, which may be blocking you from receiving the love you need from your environment or from yourself. They also enable you to find out what your dreams are and the steps you need to take to fulfill those dreams.

Useful affirmations

"The more love I allow myself to receive, the more love I have to give."

"My life is filled with love and joy."

"There is an endless source of love all around me. All I need to do is open myself up to it and receive it."

"I now allow myself to follow my own dreams. I am worth it."

Part VII

Therapies

Acupressure

This is a form of pressure point therapy (as are reflexology and shiatzu). **Acupressure** uses the same points as acupuncture to stimulate healing.

Aromatherapy

Essential oils of plants have been used since ancient times for their medicinal properties and ability to affect our moods.

For more information contact:
Aromatherapy Organisations Council
PO Box 19834, London SE25 6WS, UK. Tel. 0208 251 7912
www.aocuk.net

The National Association for Holistic Aromatherapy
4509 Interlake Ave. N., #233, Seattle, WA 98103-6773, USA. Tel. 206-547-2164
www.naha.org

Ayurvedic Medicine

This is an ancient form of medicine, with a detailed and complete medical system that aims to unite the mind, body and spirit and in this way promote healing. Ayurvedic medicine believes that nothing functions in isolation and where there is imbalance, illness will manifest. It teaches that the universe is made up of five elements—ether (space), air, fire, earth and water—and that the human body is made up of a combination of these. Ayurveda (means wisdom of life) originated over 3000 years ago in India. It shares many of its roots with Tibetan medicine and has some similarities with Chinese medicine.

For more information contact:
Dr Shantha Godagama, The Hale Clinic
7 Park Crescent, London W1N 3HE, UK. Tel. 0870-167 6667
www.ayurveda.co.uk

The National Institute of Ayurvedic Medicine
584 Milltown Road, Brewster, NY 10509, USA. Tel. 845-278-8700
www.niam.com

Chinese Medicine

This ancient form of medicine teaches that qi energy (life energy) surrounds everything and acts as the driving force in life. We all have qi in our bodies and an illness occurs when there is a blockage of qi. Disharmony of this qi triggers symptoms of disease or imbalance. It is an ancient form of medicine that goes back over 2000 years. It has many similarities with both ayurvedic and Tibetan medicine. They all believe that nothing functions in isolation and where there is an imbalance, illness will manifest. They teach that the universe is made up of five elements and that the human body is also made up of a combination of these.

For more information contact:
British Acupuncture Council
63 Jeddo Road, London, UK. Tel. 0208 735 0400
www.acupuncture.org.uk

Samra University of Oriental Medicine
3000 S. Robertson Blvd., 4th Floor, Los Angeles CA 90034, USA. Tel. 310-202-6444
www.samra.edu

Chiropractic

This therapy is a mixture of a philosophy, a science and an art. At the heart of its philosophy is the idea of the correlation between body structure and function in health and disease. The science includes the physical, chemical and biological sciences related to the maintenance of health and well-being, and how to prevent, alleviate and cure disease processes. The art is found in how each individual practitioner applies the philosophy and the science through the use of manual treatment. It has many similarities with osteopahty, but the treatment may vary slightly. As a general rule, chiropractors focus mainly on manipulation of joints. (see **Osteopathy**)

For more information contact:
General Chiropractic Council
Blagrave Street, Reading, Berks RG11QB, London, UK. Tel. 0208-950 5950
www.gcc-uk.org

Council of Chiropractic Education
8049 North 85th Way, Scottsdale, AZ 85258-4321, USA. Tel. 480-443-8877
www.cce-usa.org

Cranial Osteopathy

Cranial Osteopathy is a highly skilled and gentle type of osteopathic treatment that encourages the release of stresses and strains throughout the body, not just the head. It places special attention on the skull, the sacrum, the musculoskeletal structure, the meningeal sheaths, the cerebrospinal fluid, the fascia (connective tissue), the nervous system, the organs, bone marrow and fluids. All cranial osteopaths are qualified osteopaths with a minimum of four years full-time training.

Healing

Healing is one of the most natural ways of helping someone restore well-being. A mother does it automatically when her child has fallen and hurt himself. She immediately gives him a cuddle and kisses the injured area. When a friend is upset you instinctively give her a hug and she feels better. This is because with your intent to help another person you transfer a loving, healing, life energy force to the person. This life energy is all around us, as well as inside our physical, emotional, mental and spiritual bodies. When we are out of balance we are unable

to access this life energy effectively, and ill health, emotional turbulence and mental confusion manifest. This is where the healer is able to help. By channeling this universal life energy, the healer is able to restore and balance the energy and life force within the patient. Different types of healing are used throughout the world, such as higher-self therapy, Reiki, chakra healing, shamanistic healing, faith healing, aura healing, prayer healing and spiritual healing.

For more information contact:
National Federation of Spiritual Healers
Old Manor Farm Studio, Church Street, Sunbury-on-Thames, Middlesex TW16 6RG, UK. Tel. 01932-783164
www.nfsh.org.uk

First Spiritual Temple
The Ayer Institute, 16 Monmouth Street, Brookline, MA, 02446-5605 USA. Tel. 617-566-7639
www.fst.org

Homeopathy

Homeopathy is an effective, scientific system of healing which is based on the theory that 'like cures like', or 'that which made me sick can heal me'. Homeopathy views symptoms as signs of disharmony and believes that you treat the whole person not the symptoms.

For more information contact:
The Society of Homeopaths
4a Artizan Road, Northampton NN1 4HU, UK. Tel. 01604-621400
www.homeopathy-soh.com

National Center for Homeopathy
801 N. Fairfax Street, Suite 306, Alexandria, VA 22314, USA. Tel. 877-624-6613
www.homeopathic.org

Hypnosis

We all experience a light trance state every time our conscious mind becomes engrossed in something and it stops chattering. During those moments when you relax your conscious mind, you are in deep contact with your unconscious mind. Every time you meditate and visualize, you are in a light hypnotic trance. Most hypnotherapists use this light trance state for their treatments (not like the stage hypnotists) and you are in full control during the session.

For more information contact:

British Hypnotherapy Association
67 Upper Berkley Street, London WIH7DH, UK. Tel. 0207 723 4443
www.hypnotherapy-association.org

American Board of Hypnotherapy
615 Piikoi Street, Suite 501, Honolulu, HI 96814 USA. Tel. 808-596-7765
www.hypnosis.com

Kinesiology

Kinesiology is both a diagnostic tool and a treatment method. It uses muscle-testing as a way of finding out if the body's energy system and electrical flow have been disrupted. It believes that such a disruption shows up as a muscle weakness, and the treatment is then aimed towards rebalancing this.

For more information contact:

Middle England School of Kinesiology
81 Lancashire Street, Leicester LE47AF, UK. Tel. 0116 266 1962
www.naturalhealthdirect.com

Touch For Health Kinesiology Association
PO Box 392, New Carlisle, OH 45344-0392, USA. Tel. 800-466-8342
www.tfhka.org

Meditation and Visualisation

Meditation and visualisation have been used for thousands of years in all cultures around the world as a way to promote healing of the body, mind and spirit. It is the most natural state there is. Anytime you lose yourself in daydreaming you are effectively meditating and visualizing…it is something your brain takes to very easily.

Meditation is a peaceful state where your chattering mind (the conscious mind) becomes still, so that you can connect with your unconscious mind and spiritual self. Visualisation has long been used to aid in improving and restoring complete well-being. Through the power of the mind we send out powerful thought energies, which start to create our reality. Thoughts are made of fast-moving energy, while matter is more dense and slow-moving energy. It may appear as if our thoughts have nothing to do with our immediate reality, but every thing once started as a thought. This is the power of visualisation.

For more information contact:

Vipassana Meditation Centre
Dhamma Dipa, Harewood End, Hereford HR28JS, UK. Tel. 01989 730234
www.dipa.dhamma.org

Vipassana Meditation Center
Dhamma Dhara, 386 Colrain-Shelburne Road, Shelburne, MA 01370, USA. Tel. 413-625-2160
www.dhamma.org

Naturopathy

This is a philosophy, a science and a practice that aims to promote and maintain health and well-being within the body, mind and spirit through stimulating and assisting the inner healing power. It believes the body is able to heal itself provided it is given the appropriate support. It sees the patient as a whole being—body, mind and spirit—therefore it will always attempt to find the true root cause of illness, and not just treat the symptoms. Treatment consists of advice on diet, supplementation and herbs; neuro-musculo-skeletal adjustments to stimulate the mechanical health of the body; hydrotherapy; and advice on how to improve emotional, mental and spiritual well-being.

Dietary sources of Vitamins

• Vitamin A - liver, fish liver oils, butter, cheese, eggs, carrots, green leafy vegetables
• Vitamin B1 - whole grains, seeds, beans, nuts, fish
• Vitamin B2 - dairy products, eggs, liver, fish, nuts, leafy vegetables, broccoli
• Vitamin B3 - dairy products, liver, fish, brown rice, wholemeal bread and nuts
• Vitamin B5 - liver, kidney, fish, nuts, beans, whole grains
• Vitamin B6 - whole grains, nuts, seeds, fish, avocados, soy beans, oats
• Vitamin B12 - meat, fish, poultry, eggs, dairy products, miso, tempeh
• Biotin - liver, eggs, sardines, nuts, beans, soy products
• Folic acid - wheatgerm, beans, green leafy vegetables, asparagus, nuts, yeast extract
• Vitamin C - fruits (especially citrus), berries, kiwi, papaya; vegetables (such as tomatoes and all dark green vegetables)
• Vitamin D - it is made by the skin in response to sunlight, but is also found in food sources, such as milk, yoghurt, eggs, butter, fatty fish
• Vitamin E - wheatgerm, nuts, seeds, soy beans, whole grains, olives, avocados
• Vitamin K - green leafy vegetables

Dietary sources of nutrients related to vitamins

• Co-enzyme Q10 - organ meats, egg yolk, milkfat, whole grains
• Bioflavonoids - the white rind in citrus fruit, vegetables, honey

Dietary sources of Minerals

• Boron - alfalfa, almonds, soy beans, cabbage, peas, raisins, apples
• Calcium - sesame seeds, tofu, green leafy vegetables, dairy products, cooked bones as in canned sardines
• Chromium - red meat, liver, seafood, whole grains, pulses, cheese
• Copper - organ meat, seafood, nuts, seeds
• Fluoride - seafood, meat, tea
• Iodine - seaweed, seafood, mackerel, haddock, live yoghurt, iodized salt
• Iron - dark green leafy vegetables, dark cocoa, dried fruits, molasses, red meat
• Magnesium - whole grains, green leafy vegetables, wheatgerm, dried apricots, soy beans, almonds, cashews
• Manganese - whole grains, rice bran, nuts, wheatgerm, black tea, ginger, pulses, fruits, vegetables
• Phosphorus - whole grains, fish, meats, nuts
• Potassium - bananas, dried fruits, pumpkin seeds, almonds, soy beans, potatoes, green leafy vegetables, fish, avocado
• Selenium - Brazil nuts, cashews, tuna, soy beans, seafood, meat, whole grains, avocados, lentils
• Sodium - We get too much sodium through our diet, since it is present in all processed food. Even if you never eat any processed food, there is more than enough sodium present in vegetables.

• Sulphur - meat, fish, eggs, beans, nuts
• Zinc - seafood, pumpkin seeds, sunflower seeds, fish, popcorn, wheatgerm, meat, eggs, cheese

Hydrotherapy treatments

Cold treatments are helpful for inflammation. Place an ice pack on the painful area for five to ten minutes, sit in a cold bath, or take a cold shower.

Hot and cold treatments stimulate circulation. Apply heat for three minutes, then apply cold for one minute. Repeat. This can also be done in the shower by using flannels or washcloths, or in a 'sitz bath' (especially good for pelvic problems): partially fill a bathtub with warm water, and also place a large container with ice cold water. First sit in the warm bath with your feet in the ice cold water, then sit in the container of cold water with your feet in the warm bath.

Epsom salts baths are wonderful for detoxing. Soak for 20 minutes in a luke-warm bath filled with Epsom salts. Then shower with warm water and then with cold water. Rub yourself dry vigorously with a towel.

Steam inhalants help clear congestion. Put the desired ingredients, such as Olbas Oil, various aromatherapy oils or herbs, in a bowl of hot water. Place a large towel over your head and lean over the bowl. Breathe in the steam, so you fill your lungs completely with the qualities from the ingredients.

Packs and compresses

Castor oil packs are used for detoxing. Soak a cloth in heated castor oil, making sure it is not too hot. Place the cloth over the desired area (usually the liver to aid in detoxification). Then wrap with cling film and place a warm towel around everything. You can also use a towel wrapped around a hot water bottle, or use a heating pad. Rest with the pack on for up to one hour. Use baking soda to wash off the oil afterwards, as ordinary soap will not remove it.

Compresses are also used for detoxing. Take a soft cloth soaked in a hot or a cold infusion of the desired ingredient and place on the afflicted area.

For more information contact:
British Naturopathic Association
Goswell House, 2 Goswell Road, Somerset BA 160JH, UK. Tel. 0870 745 6984
www.naturopaths.org.uk

American Naturopathic Medical Association (ANMA)
P.O Box 96273, Las Vegas, Nevada 89193, USA. Tel. (702)897-7053
www.anma.com

Neuro-Linguistic Programming (NLP)

NLP is often described as an attitude and a methodology that leaves behind a trail of techniques. The attitude is a sense of curiosity, which enables you to discover new ways of thinking. The methodology is a tool box of techniques designed to create maximum, specific, positive changes and results enabling you to live the life of your dreams and experience well-being on all levels—physical, emotional, mental and spiritual. It does all this by allowing you to take charge of the most amazing computer ever created—your brain.

At the core of NLP is the knowledge that we only perceive our outside reality according to our inner world. So your experience is always just your own, and it only has the meaning which you attach to it.

Since NLP allows you to let go of unwanted states and behaviours and enables you to take control over your mind so that you are able to achieve resourceful, positive states and create desired behaviours and outcomes, it can benefit anyone, as long as they are ready to change.

For more information contact:
The Performance Partnership, Rosedale House, Rosedale Road London TW92SZ, UK. Tel. 0208 992 9523
www.performancepartnership.com

The Well-Being Partnership, Oxford, UK. Tel. 0845 838 5517
www.wellbeingpartnership.com

American Board of NLP
615 Piikoi Street, Suite 501, Honolulu, Hawaii 96814, USA. Tel. 808-596-7765
www.nlp.com

Osteopathy

This therapy is a mixture of a philosophy, a science and an art. At the heart of its philosophy is the idea of the correlation between body structure and function in health and disease. The science includes the physical, chemical and biological sciences related to the maintenance of health and well-being, and how to prevent, alleviate and cure disease processes. The art is found in how each individual practitioner applies the philosophy and the science is expressed through the use of manual treatment. It has many similarities with chiropractic, but the treatment may vary slightly. As a general rule, osteopaths focus on manipulation and mobilising of joints and releasing of muscular, visceral and fascial tension. (see **Chiropractic**)

For more information contact:
The General Osteopathic Council
Osteopathy House, 176 Tower Bridge Road, London SE13LU, UK. Tel. 0207 357 6655
www.osteopathy.org.uk
American Academy of Osteopathy
3500 DePauw Blvd., Suite 1080, Indianapolis, IN 46268, USA. Tel. 317-879-1881
www.academyofosteopathy.org

Pilates

Pilates is a system of body conditioning that involves strengthening and stretching exercises to improve the function of the entire system. Pilates believes in training the mind and body to work as an integrated unit to produce physical and overall fitness. The main principles are: concentration to focus the mind and body on a specific area; control of muscle in order to avoid injury; centering, involving attention to the 'powerhouse' muscles of the mid-section, abdomen, lower back, buttocks and hips; fluidity, emphasising smooth graceful movements; precision, to perform each movement purposefully and efficiently; integration, to use the body as it was intended, as a whole; and most importantly, breathing, in order to cleanse the circulation and facilitate or stabilise the body.

For more information contact:
Polestar Pilates UK
PO Box 42704, London N2OWE, UK. Tel. 0870 246 0280
www.polestareducation.co.uk

Balanced Body Pilates USA
7500 14th Ave., Suite 23, Sacramento, CA 95820, USA. Tel. 916-458-2838
www.pilates.com

Reflexology

This is a form of pressure point therapy (as are acupressure and shiatzu). Reflexology is based on the belief that the feet and the hands mirror the body, and by stimulating specific reflex points, different organs and body systems can be affected.

For more information contact:
Association of Reflexologists, 27 Old Gloucester Street, London WC1N3XX, UK. Tel. 08705 673320
www.aor.org.uk

Reflexology Association of America
79 Hudson Road, Bolton, MA 01740, USA.
Tel. 978-779-0255
www.reflexology-usa.org

Shiatzu

This is a form of pressure point therapy (as are acupressure and reflexology). Shiatzu is the Japanese version of acupressure.

Tibetan Medicine

This is an ancient form of medicine that aims to unite mind, body and spirit to promote healing. According to Tibetan medicine the body is the physical expression of mental energies generated by the brain. Therefore, it helps the patient to understand the root cause of an illness and holds the illness both in the mind and the body. This is why it aims to help people change their behavioural and thought patterns, even if the injury appears to be of a physical nature, such as a broken arm. Tibetan Medicine is practised by both Tibetan Buddhist Medicine and the more ancient form of Tibetan Dur Bön Medicine. Dur Bön is a shamanistic medicine and religion, which dates back some 17000 years, and it was the original religion of the people in Tibet. Both types of Tibetan medicine search for compassion, wisdom and virtue, and believe that in order to grow spiritually you must first increase your personal energy and vitality. They feel that skilful use of thought energy is the key to empowerment. Through mastering anger, envy, jealousy, greed, lust, arrogance, selfishness, careless actions and thoughts we are able to let go of our reactions to other peoples actions and thoughts. In this way we master the ability to think true original thoughts, which is one of the most powerful energy resources we all have. Tapping in to this powerful source we are able to create happiness and well-being.

For more information contact:
Christopher Hansard, The Eden Medical Centre, 63a Kings Road, London SW3 4NT, UK. Tel. 0207 881 5800
www.edenmedicalcentre.com
The Bon Foundation, PO Box 826, Exeter, NH 03833-0826, USA. Tel. 603-778-6997
www.bonfoundation.org

Visualisation

see Meditation and Visualisation

Yoga

Yoga is a science of life; a spiritual approach to living that had its roots in India many thousands of years ago. Yoga has several branches, or paths to follow depending on the individual, such as Hatha yoga, Iyengar yoga and Ashtanga yoga. They each involve physical postures (asanas) and breathing control methods (pranayama), and all of them originally developed from classical Hatha yoga. Each has a different emphasis.

Titles such as 'power yoga' are used increasingly in modern times but it should not be forgotten that yoga is primarily a spiritual way of living and the body is only part of its all-encompassing scope of practice. The word 'yoga' means to 'yoke' (to join), and it is the very purpose of yoga to reunite the individual self with the Absolute (pure consciousness).

For more information contact:
Sivananda Yoga Vedanta Centre
51 Felsham Road, London SW15 1AZ, UK.
Tel: 020 8780 0160
www.sivananda.org/london

International Sivenanda Yoga Vedanta Centres
Sivananda Ashram Yoga Ranch
PO Box 195, Budd Road, Woodbourne, NY 12788 USA. Tel. 845-436-6492
www.sivananda.org

Bibliography and References

Bibliography

Balaskas, Janet and Yehudi Gordon. *Pregnancy and Birth*. London: A Little Brown Book, 1992.

Berkow, Robert, ed. *The Merck Manual*. Rahway, NJ: Merck & Co. Inc., 1993.

Boucher, Ian, ed. *The Index of Differential Diagnosis*. Oxford: Reed Educational and Professional Publishing Ltd., 1996.

Brandon, Bays. *The Journey*. London: Element, 2003.

Carreiro, Jane. *An Osteopathic Approach to Children*. London: Churchill Livingstone, 2003.

Chopra, Deepak. *Ageless Body, Timeless Mind*. New York: Harmony Books, 1993.

Clayden, Graham, and Tom Lissauer. *Illustrated Textbook of Paediatrics*. London: Mosby International Ltd., 2002.

Crawford Adams, John. *An Outline of Orthopaedics*. London: Churchill Livingstone, 1990.

Epstein, Owen. *Clinical Examination*. London: Gower Medical Publishing, 1992.

Gawain, Shakti. *Creative Visualisations*. California: New World Library, 1995.

Gawain, Shakti. *Reflections in the Light*. California: New World Library, 1988.

Godogama, Shanta. *The Handbook of Ayurveda*. London: Kyle Cathie Ltd, 1997.

Gray, John. *How To Get What You Want and Want What You Have*. London: Ebury Press, 1999.

Hansard, Christopher. *The Tibetan Art of Positive Thinking*. London: Hodder and Stoughton, 2003.

Hay, Louise. *The Power Is Within You*. London: Eden Grove Editions, 1991.

Hay, Louise. *You Can Heal Your Life*. London: Eden Grove Editions, 1988.

Jampolsky, Gerald. *Love is the Answer*. New York: Bantam Books, 1990.

Kubler-Ross, Elizabeth and David Kessler. *Life Lessons*. London: Simon & Schuster UK Ltd., 2000.

Lama, Dalai. *The Art of Happiness*. London: Hodder and Stoughton, 1999.

Linenger, Schuyler. *The Natural Pharmacy*. California: Health Notes Inc., 1999.

McTaggart, Lynne, ed. *The Medical Desk Reference*. London, 2000.
Mortimore, Denise. *Nutritional Healing*. Dorset: Element Books Ltd. 1998.

Murray, Michael. *Encyclopaedia of Nutritional Supplements*. California: Prima Publishing, 1996.

Murray, Michael and Joseph Pizzorno. *Encyclopaedia of Natural Medicine*. California: Prima Publishing, 1998.

Myss, Caroline. *The Anatomy of the Spirit*. London: Bantam Books, 1996.

Northage, Ivy. *Spiritual Realisations*. London: College of Psychic Studies, 1995.

Read, Alan and John Jones. *Essential Medicine*. London: Churchill Livingstone, 1993.

Robbins, Anthony. *Unlimited Power*. New York: Fireside, 1997.

Roman, Sanya. *Living with Joy*. California: HJ Kramer Inc. 1986.

Roman, Sanya. *Spiritual Growth*. California: HJ Kramer Inc. 1989.

Shapiro, Debbie. *The Bodymind Work Book*. Dorset: Element Books Ltd., 1990.

Shaw, Non. *Herbalism, an Illustrated Guide*. Dorset: Element Books Ltd., 1998.

Schuman, Helen and William Thetford. *A Course in Miracles*. California: Foundation for Inner Peace, 1992.

Thurston, Mark. *The Great Teachings of Edgar Cayce*. Virginia: Association for Research and Enlightenment, 1996.

Trattler, Ross. *Better Health Through Natural Healing*. New York: McGraw-Hill Book Company, 1985.

Vogel, Alfred. *The Nature Doctor*. Edinburgh: Mainstream Publishing Company Ltd., 1989.

Walsch, Neale Donald. *Conversations with God*. London: Hodder and Stoughton, 1997.

Ward, Robert, ed. *The Foundations of Osteopathic Medicine*. Maryland, USA: Williams & Wilkins, 1997.

Williamson, Marianne. *Return to Love*. London: Thorsons, 1992.

Yogananda, Paramahansa. *Where There is Light*. California: Self Realisation Fellowship, 1988.

References

(1) R. Rimoldi, F. Ginesu, and R. Giura, "The use of Bromelain in Pneumological Therapy", Drugs Exp Clin Res 4(1978): 55–66.

(2) J.C Stiles et al., J Applied Nutr 47 (1995): 96–102.

(3) M.C Martin, J.E. Block, S.D Sanchez et al.,"Menopause without symptoms: The Endocrinology among Rural Mayan Indians", Am J Obstet Gynecol 168 (1993): 1939–45

(4) J. Siegel, Ann Allergy 32 (1974): 127–30 and C.Andre et al., Ann Allergy 51 (1983): 325–8

(5) 'Live right 4 your type' by Dr. P J. D'Adamo.

(6) J. Jarnerot et al, Scand J Gastroenterol. 18 (1983): 999–1002

(7) A.J Levi, Gut 26 (1985): 985–8

(8) L. Demling Hepato Gastroent. 41 (1994): 549–51

(9) R. Nanda et al., Gut 30(1989): 1099–1104

(10) D. Gertner and J. Powell-Tuck, Practitioner 238 (1994): 499–504

(11) V. Jones et al., Lancet ii (1982): 1115–18

(12) BMJ, 1985; 291:109

(13) AM Fitness 1993; 11:24–6

(14) Petersdorf, R., Harrison's Principles of Internal Medicine, 10th Ed., McGraw-Hill, 1983

(15) The Medical Desk Reference, 2000: 172

(16) G. Drner, A. Mohnike, and H. Thoelke, "Further evidence for the dependance of diabetes prevalence on nutrition in prenatal life", Exp Clin Endocrinol 84 (1984): 129–33

(17) R.D.G Leslie and R.B Eliott, Diabetes 43 (1994): 843–50

(18) Eur J Clin Nutr 1988; 42:51–4; Eur J Clin Nutr, 1990; 44:301–6

(19) Am J Clin Nutr, 1990; 52:675–81

(20) Arch Intern Med, 2000; 160:1009–13

(21) Curr Probs in Pharm, Feb 1994 quoted in Medical Desk Reference 2000

(22) H. Trowell, D. Burkitt and K. Heaton, Dietary fibre, fibre depleted foods and disease, London, UK: Academic Press 1985

(23) Br J Surg 65 (1978): 291–92; Dis Colon Rectum 25 (1982): 454–56

(24) JAMA, 1995; 274:1526–33, Clinical Investigator 1993; 71:993–8

(25) Irish J Med Science;1995;164 Suppl 15: 51A

(26) J Amer Col Nutr, 1985;4:195–206, Magnesium Bulletin,1981;3: 165–77

(27) S.S Gottlieb et al., J Am Coll Cardiol 16(1990): 827–31

(28) M. Brodsky et al., Am J Cardio 73(1994): 1227–9

(29) C. Hofman-Bang et al., J Am Coll Cardiol 19 (1992): 216A

(30) Morisco, et al, Clin Investig 71 (suppl.8) (1993): S134–6

(31) T. Oda etal, Jap Circ J 48(1984): 1387

(32) K. Folkers et al, Proc Natl. Acad Sci 82 (1985): 901

(33) H. Leuchtgens; Fortschr Med 111 (1993): 352–4

(34) Hafter, Hertha, 'Phosphates in food as a cause of behavioural disturbances in teenage delinquents. Heidelberg, kriminalistik verlag, 1979

(35) G. Hussey et al, N Engl J Med 323 (1990): 160–4

(36) R. Brayton et al, NEJM 282 (1970): 123–8

(37) M. Irvin et al. Biol. Psych.27(1990): 22–30

(38) M. Alexander et al. Immunol Letters 9 (1985): 221–4

(39) S.N Meydani et al, JAMA 277 (1997): 1380–6

(40) H. Hasselbach et al, Acta Pedriatr 85 (1996): 1029–32

(41) N.M Norman and K.S.M Lancet 2 (1985): 11–13

(42) H. Ronningen, N.Langeland Acta Ortop.Scand 50(1979): 169–74

(43) WDDTY Volume 5 No 5

(44) H. Muller-Fassbender et al.,'Osteoarthritis cartilage 2' (1994): 61–69

(45) L.C Rovati et al., Osteoarthritis cartilage 2 (suppl.1) (1994): 56

(46) I.R Reid et al., Am J Med 98 (1995): 331–35

(47) I.R Reid Am J Med Sci 312 (1996): 278–86 and Osteoporosis int 7 (1997): 23–28

(48) G. Stendig-Lundberg et al., Magnesium Res 6 (1993): 155–63

(49) D.L Scott et al., Lancet 1(1989): 1108–11

(50) Acta Endocrinologica, 1993: 128:293–6

(51) J Endocrinol Invest, 1994, 17:23–7

(52) J Clin Endocrinol Metab, 1983, 57: 859–62

(53) Clin Endocrinol. (Oxford), 1984;21: 163–72

(54) R. Ryan, Headache 7 (1967): 13–7

(55) C.A Silagy and H.A.Neil, J Hypertens 12(4)(1994): 463–8

(56) J.A Simon. J Am Coll Nutr 11 (1992):107–25

(57) E.B Schmidt and J. Dyerberg, Drugs 47 (1994): 405–24

(58) L.J Appel et al., Arch Intern Med 153 (1993): 1429–38

(59) P. Langsjoen et al., Mol Aspects Med 15 (suppl)(1994): S265–72

(60) S. Gregersen et al., Eur J Clin Nutr 46 (1992): 301–1

(61) V.A Koivisto et al., Journal of Internal Medicine 233 (1993): 145–53

(62) R.L Swank et al., "Multiple Sclerosis in Rural Norway": NEJM 246 (1952) 721–8

(63) Frisk, Per, Hälsa, nr.2 (February 2005): 69

This book is lovingly dedicated to my two wonderful daughters,
Erika and Natasha.
May you always continue to shine your inner light, love
and happiness wherever you go and know deep within your Souls
how beautiful and amazing you are.

If you would like to know more about the work of **Cissi Williams**,
or want to participate in Well-Being workshops,
train with her personally or have private sessions,
please feel free to call 0845 838 5517
or visit **www.nordiclightinstitute.com**

For further information about the Findhorn Foundation and the Findhorn Community, please contact:

Findhorn Foundation

The Visitors Centre
The Park, Findhorn IV36 3TZ, Scotland, UK
tel 01309 690311
enquiries@findhorn.org
www.findhorn.org

For a complete Findhorn Press catalogue, please contact:

Findhorn Press

305a The Park, Findhorn
Forres IV36 3TE
Scotland, UK
tel 01309 690582
fax 01309 690036
info@findhornpress.com
www.findhornpress.com